Putting Patients First

Susan B. Frampton, Laura Gilpin, Patrick A. Charmel, Editors

Putting Patients First

Designing and Practicing Patient-Centered Care

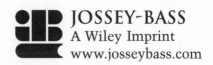
JOSSEY-BASS
A Wiley Imprint
www.josseybass.com

Published by Jossey-Bass
A Wiley Imprint
989 Market Street, San Francisco, CA 94103-1741   www.josseybass.com

Jossey-Bass books and products are available through most bookstores. To contact Jossey-Bass directly call our Customer Care Department within the U.S. at 800-956-7739, outside the U.S. at 317-572-3986 or fax 317-572-4002.

Jossey-Bass also publishes its books in a variety of electronic formats. Some content that appears in print may not be available in electronic books.

Library of Congress Cataloging-in-Publication Data

    Putting patients first : designing and practicing patient-centered care
/ Susan B. Frampton, Laura Gilpin, Patrick A. Charmel, editors.
    p. ; cm.
    Includes bibliographical references and index.
    ISBN 0-7879-6412-3 (alk. paper)
    1. Medical personnel and patient. 2. Hospital care. [DNLM: 1. Patient-Centered Care—methods. 2. Patient-Centered Care—trends. W 84.5 P993 2003] I. Frampton, Susan B. II. Gilpin, Laura, 1950- III. Charmel, Patrick A.
    R727.3.P88 2003
    610.69'6—dc21   2003002588

Printed in the United States of America
FIRST EDITION
HB Printing   10 9 8 7 6 5 4

Contents

Part One: Nine Elements of Patient-Centered Care

Acknowledgments

We would like to express our deepest gratitude to Planetree's founder, Angelica Thieriot, for her extraordinary vision of health care's highest potential, for her courage in believing that transformation was possible, and for her passion in bringing that vision into reality.

We are indebted to so many, who, over Planetree's twenty-five-year history, have helped to nurture, shape, and guide that vision to become the national organization it is today. We are especially grateful to Planetree's founding board of directors, whose names are listed below, and to many others, including Patricia Ryan Phelan, Robin Orr, Rochelle Perrine Schmalz, and Tracey Cosgrove. And we will always treasure the memory of Roslyn Lindheim.

We would also like to extend our gratitude to the many pioneers from our initial model sites, especially John Aird, Bob Brueckner, Randy Carter, Candace Ford Gray, Steven Horowitz, JoAnn Iocobellis, Bobby Kimball, Allan Komarek, John Liu, Deborah Matza, William Powanda, Carol Rich, Marc Schweitzer, Jacque Scott, Mark Scott, Aubrey Serfling, Bruce Spivey, Ellie Trondsend, Carol Wahl, and Lynn Werdal. We are also grateful to those who have helped to articulate the vision and inspire others, including Leland Kaiser, Bill Moyers, Tom Peters, Roger Ulrich, Bruce Arneill, Kirk Hamilton, F. Nicholas Jacobs, Donald Berwick, and Susan Edgman-Levitan.

Planetree has received grants and contributions from many organizations over the past twenty-five years; they have made Planetree's work possible. We are grateful to all of them and would like to acknowledge especially The Henry J. Kaiser Family Foundation and The San Francisco Foundation, whose support made the establishment of the original Planetree model site possible.

We would also like to thank the members of the Planetree Alliance and the hundreds of nurses, physicians, administrators, managers, librarians, volunteers, and others who, through their work each day, continue to advance the philosophy and principles of patient-centered, family-centered, and community-centered care.

Thanks especially to the patients themselves, who, throughout the years, have so generously shared their stories and perceptions with us, continually inspiring us to expand the vision of what is possible in health care. We would also like to thank those like-minded individuals and organizations, who, through their ongoing work, are helping to make the vision we all share a reality.

We would also like to acknowledge recent members of the Planetree board of directors—in particular, Mary Pittman for her assistance in launching this book project. Finally, we would like to thank the supportive staff members of the Planetree national office for their help with the preparation of this manuscript, and, in particular, Marie Sullivan, Planetree assistant, who has the patience of a saint.

The members of Planetree's founding board of directors in 1978 included Eileen Aicardi, Suzanne Arms, Joan Barbour, Stewart Brand, Rick Carlson, Don C. Creevy, Mary Crowley, Phelps Dewey, Betsy Everdell, Victoria Fay, John Gamble, Jill Goffstein, Lee Gruhn, Fred G. Hudson, Gretchen Cebrian Krinsky, Maryon Davies Lewis, Roslyn Lindheim, Cyril Magnin, Marie Manthey, Sandra Mosbacher, Stanley Parry, Patricia Ryan Phelan, David Sobel, Charles Thieriot, Jordan Wilbur, and John Williford. We are grateful to each one of them.

Susan Frampton, Laura Gilpin, and Patrick A. Charmel
The Editors

The Editors

Susan B. Frampton is executive director of Planetree. She received her B.A. in medical anthropology from Rutgers University and both her M.A. and her Ph.D. from the University of Connecticut, also in medical anthropology. Prior to her work with Planetree, she spent over twenty years at several hospitals in the New England area. Her work focused on community education, wellness and prevention, planning, and the development of integrative medicine service lines. Frampton has numerous publications, including recent chapters in *Integrating Complementary Medicine into Health Systems* (2001) and *Best Practice Leadership Champions* (forthcoming), as well as articles and interviews in *Modern Healthcare* (2002), *Complementary Health Practice Review* (2001), and *Hospitals and Health Networks* (2002). She speaks widely on cultural and organizational practices, patient-centered care, and health care consumerism.

Laura Gilpin is director of the Planetree Alliance. She holds a B.A. from Sarah Lawrence College, a master of fine arts degree from Columbia University, and a B.S. in nursing from New York University. Her involvement with Planetree began in 1985, when she worked as a staff nurse on the original Planetree Model unit at Pacific Presbyterian Medical Center in San Francisco. She then served as the first patient educator and arts coordinator.

Gilpin has published widely, including a chapter in *Managing Hospital-Based Patient Education* (1993). She has also published a book of poetry, *The Hocus-Pocus of the Universe* (1977), for which she received the Walt Whitman Award from the Academy of American Poets. She was awarded a Writer's Grant in 1981 from the National Endowment for the Arts.

Gilpin taught creative writing at the Henry Street Settlement and at the New York Public Library before becoming a registered nurse. Her nursing career includes pediatric nursing at Memorial Sloan-Kettering Cancer Center in New York and adult oncology at Pacific Presbyterian Medical Center in San Francisco (now California Pacific Medical Center).

Patrick A. Charmel is president and chief executive officer at Griffin Health Services Corporation, which is the parent organization of Planetree and Griffin Hospital. He has been associated with Griffin Hospital in Derby, Connecticut, since 1979, where he served a student internship while attending Quinnipiac College. After graduating from Quinnipiac College, he received his M.P.H. from Yale University. He is a Diplomat of the American College of Health Care Executives.

During his tenure with Griffin, Charmel has positioned the hospital as an award-winning, innovative organization. He has been recognized as an industry leader in providing personalized, humanistic, consumer-driven health care in a healing environment and for establishing an organizational culture and human resources practices that have resulted in Griffin Hospital being named to *Fortune* magazine's list of "The 100 Best Companies to Work For" in 2000, 2001, 2002, and 2003.

Charmel is a member of the board of trustees of the Connecticut Hospital Association, the board of governors of the Quinnipiac University Alumni Association, and the board of directors of the Greater Valley Chamber of Commerce. He is a corporator of the Valley United Way, and has served on many additional community and professional association boards and councils. Charmel was inducted into the Junior Achievement Free Enterprise Hall of Fame in 2002. He is the recipient of the Dean Avery Award, given by the New London Day newspaper in recognition of individual commitment to the public's right to know.

The Contributors

Bruce Arneill is founder and chair emeritus of The S/L/A/M Collaborative in Glastonbury, Connecticut, a 160-person architectural firm nationally known for health care design and a past winner of the Modern Healthcare Honor Award for a Planetree hospital. He has led the planning and design of more than fifty health care projects and is a past president of the National AIA Academy on Architecture for Health.

Arneill is currently executive director of SDA Arneill International, a consulting firm specializing in solutions, decisions, and actions for health care management, where he uses his broad range of experience in planning, design, writing, and teaching. Arneill has taught for many years at such institutions as Harvard University, the American Hospital Association, and the Group Health Association of America, as well as at the Yale School of Hospital Administration, where he is teaching an ongoing course on the management of operational issues. He has been widely published in professional journals and recently planned and wrote the latest JCAHO booklet, *Guidelines for Healthcare Planning and Design* (1996). He also wrote *Design Guidelines and Process for Planetree Facilities* (2000).

Randall Carter is the director of organizational development and strategy for Planetree. Carter's experience in developing and sustaining the patient-centered model in a variety of settings provides network members with an exceptional resource for organizational analysis, strategy, and employee development. Carter also provides consultation to facilities in the planning and creation of healing environments through physical plant changes or new construction.

Prior to joining Planetree in 2002, Carter served for eleven years as the administrative director of education and facilities, and he was an executive management team member at Mid-Columbia Medical Center (MCMC) in The Dalles, Oregon. MCMC was the first hospital to implement systemwide the Planetree philosophy of care in the United States. During Carter's tenure at MCMC, the organization was recognized in numerous health care periodicals and books, including *Turned-On Organizations* (1996) and *Patient-Focused Healing* (1993), as well as in Bill Moyer's landmark documentary series on PBS, *Healing and the Mind*.

Early in 1991, Carter developed the MCMC University program to share with employees the vision, information, and skills necessary to achieve this innovation in health care delivery. Carter has consulted and delivered programs on attitude, service, quality, teamwork, patient-centered care, and the development of healing environments to hundreds of audiences, including hospitals, physician groups, and diverse audiences outside of health care, including those in building and design, retail, software, education, broadcasting, public utilities, and government.

Susan Edgman-Levitan served initially as associate director and program manager, and later as president and CEO, for the Picker Institute, a Boston-based nonprofit research and consulting firm. Under her guidance, the Picker Institute worked with hundreds of health care institutions to design and administer patient satisfaction surveys. Edgman-Levitan's professional interests have focused on hospital- and community-based primary care, strategies to enhance individuals' ability to live productively with illness, and nontraditional approaches to illness. She currently serves as a special consultant to the Robert Wood Johnson "Pursuing Perfection in Health Care" grant programs.

Candace Ford, director of the Planetree Health Library in San Jose, California, has been a librarian for twenty-five years. Before her work with Planetree began in 1987, she worked in public libraries, and has also managed corporate and hospital libraries. As director of the second oldest Planetree library, Ford contributed to the revisions of the Planetree Classification Scheme and has given presentations at numerous national conferences. She has served as a Planetree consultant helping affiliates and other organizations start community health libraries.

Karrie Frasca-Beaulieu is an associate at the architectural firm The S/L/A/M Collaborative, nationally known for its health care design. Frasca-Beaulieu has specialized in the field of health care design for over fifteen years, has served as the lead designer for Griffin Hospital in Derby, Connecticut (a Planetree hospital), and is a past winner of the Modern Healthcare Honor Award. As an award-winning S/L/A/M team designer, she is nationally recognized for her ability to transform sterile, institutional spaces into nurturing and healing environments.

Frasca-Beaulieu is the author of several publications on the vital connection between wellness and the physical environment, and has examined the importance of design as an integral part and partner in the healing process. Her publications include "Interior Design for Ambulatory Care Facilities: How to Reduce Stress and Anxiety in Patients and Family" in the January 1999 issue of the *Journal of Ambulatory Care Management* and "Design Guidelines and Process for Planetree Facilities" (2000).

Trevor Hancock is a public health physician and health promotion consultant based in British Columbia, Canada. He has been a principal of Planetree Canada, as well as chair of the board of the Canadian Association of Physicians for the Environment. A prolific writer and speaker on the role of hospitals in community health initiatives and the promotion of environmental responsibility in health care, he has played a key role in expanding the Planetree model of care to include the promotion of healthy communities.

Rev. George Handzo received his clinical pastoral education at Yale–New Haven Hospital as well as at Lutheran Medical Center in Brooklyn, New York, and he is ordained in the Evangelical Lutheran Church in America. He is director of clinical services at The HealthCare Chaplaincy in New York City, after having been, for over twenty years, director of chaplaincy services at the Memorial Sloan-Kettering Cancer Center in New York City, a partner institution of The HealthCare Chaplaincy. Rev. Handzo is the author of a number of articles and chapters on the subject of pastoral and spiritual care, as well as the book *Health Care Chaplaincy in Oncology* (1992), which he coauthored with Laurel Burton. He is a board-certified chaplain in the Association of Professional Chaplains and is currently the association's president-elect.

Charlene Honeycutt is a director of the Advisory Board Company in Washington, D.C. She has spent eighteen years in the health care industry and has six years of consulting experience, with a focus on achieving best practices, and she has eight years of experience with system implementation and project management of clinical systems that are primarily focused on physician adoption. Prior to her work with the Advisory Board Company, she spent nine years in critical care nursing.

Steven Horowitz served as chief of cardiology and medical director of Samuels Planetree Model Unit at Beth Israel Medical Center in New York City from 1988 to 2002. He is currently chairman of the department of cardiology at the Stamford Hospital, Stamford, Connecticut. He is also a professor of medicine and nuclear medicine at New York's Albert Einstein College of Medicine.

Horowitz championed the establishment of one of the original Planetree model sites over a decade ago and has been instrumental

in creating and maintaining a patient-centered healing environment in an organization that faces monumental operational challenges. He speaks internationally on his experiences as a cardiologist
working to personalize and demystify the hospital experience.
Horowitz serves as a national Planetree board member and consultant, and he has worked with the medical staffs of many Planetree
affiliates to achieve greater understanding and physician support for
patient-centered care.

Leland Kaiser is president of Kaiser Consulting in Brighton, Colorado, and cofounder of the Kaiser Institute, an advanced fel-
lowship program for health professionals. He is a faculty member
of the Estes Park Institute and the American College of Physician Executives and also holds an appointment as associate professor in the Executive Program in Health Administration,
Graduate School of Business at the University of Colorado at
Denver.

Dr. Kaiser is a healthcare futurist, an intuitive, an executive
coach, a community organizer, and an organizational consultant.
He is a pioneer in many emerging areas of health care including the
healthier communities movement, the development of integrative
medicine, electronic teaching technologies, the use of nonlinear
brain processes in management, and the role of spirituality in the
future of medicine. He is the author of more than two hundred
monographs, journal articles, and videotapes.

David Katz is associate clinical professor of public health and medicine and director of medical studies in public health at the Yale
University School of Medicine. He is also a board-certified specialist in both internal medicine and preventive medicine.

Katz is director of the Centers for Disease Control and Prevention–
funded Yale-Griffin Prevention Research Center, where he oversees
numerous studies of chronic disease prevention. He is also founder
and director of the Integrative Medicine Center at Griffin Hospital,

which provides dual allopathic and naturopathic care to patients in a unique model of consensus decision making.

Author of more than forty scientific papers and six books to date, Katz speaks frequently throughout the United States and abroad on topics related to disease prevention and health promotion.

Allan Komarek is the executive director of Delano Regional Medical Center (DRMC) in Delano, California, and was instrumental in bringing Planetree to the medical center in 1989. As vice president of Patient Care Enterprises, he began the implementation process on DRMC's fifty-nine-bed long-term care wing. The special care unit has become the model for subacute care in California. Despite a change in administration, the unit has continued to have a low staff turnover: 85 percent of the original staff from 1989 remain. The unit has been renovated to include a kitchen, garden, library, and stained glass windows. Programs include coma stimulation, reading to patients, care partners, and aroma therapy. Their pets include birds, rabbits, cats, and fish. They also have a strong spirituality component.

Before returning to DRMC as executive director, Komarek served as chief nursing officer at Sierra Vista Regional Medical Center in San Luis Obispo, California, and he also served as chief operating officer at Alexian Brothers Hospital in San Jose, California.

Kathy Reinke is a registered dietitian and a certified diabetes educator. As the dietary department manager at Shawano Medical Center in Shawano, Wisconsin, she has had the opportunity to plan and develop a wide variety of nutrition programs for patients and the community. Under her direction, the hospital received the Go with the Grain Gold Award in a national whole grain promotion contest through General Mills.

Reinke is a member of the American Dietetic Association, the American Society for Healthcare Food Service Administrators, the Wisconsin Dietetic Association, and several professional practice groups. She credits her mom and grandmother with instilling in her a clear understanding of the nurturing aspects of food, and she plans to continue that tradition with her family.

Carol Ryczek is the community relations manager at Shawano Medical Center. She is also a member of the Wisconsin Health Care Public Relations and Marketing Society and has been involved in coordinating and promoting community education programs for fifteen years. Ryczek has earned awards in writing and photography, and, with a group of colleagues, she was recognized for a children's wellness education program.

Michele Spatz is currently director of the Planetree Health Resource Center, a community-based consumer health library located in The Dalles, Oregon. She completed the Medical Symptom Reduction Training Program at the Center for Training in Mind/Body Medicine, Mind/Body Medical Institute of Harvard Medical School/ Deaconess Hospital, Boston, Massachusetts, during the summer of 1996. Since then, Spatz has developed and taught many stress reduction courses through the Center for Mind and Body Medicine at Mid-Columbia Medical Center. She also teaches two accredited continuing education courses for the Medical Library Association, writes a monthly health column, publishes professionally on issues related to health information for the public, serves as column editor for a quarterly professional journal, and is a member of the URAC Health Web Site Accreditation Committee.

Phyllis Stoneburner is currently the vice president for patient care services at Warren Memorial Hospital in Front Royal, Virginia, and she is responsible for the overall management of the patient care services department, including the intensive care unit, the medical-surgical-telemetry unit, the Women's Care Center, the Lynn Care Center, and subacute rehabilitation (totaling 132 beds). Stoneburner leads the steering committee for the implementation of the

Planetree model of health care at Warren Memorial Hospital, which was recognized as one of the "fifteen hospitals with heart" by the AARP in its July/August 2001 issue of *Modern Maturity* magazine.

Dianne Storby joined Mid-Columbia Medical Center (MCMC) in 1997 and is currently vice president of performance and quality systems at MCMC. Storby was appointed director of MCMC's Center for Mind and Body Medicine in 1998. Under Storby's care and guidance, massage therapy has blossomed at MCMC.

Roger Ulrich is professor of architecture at Texas A&M University and serves as director of the Center for Health Systems and Design, an interdisciplinary center housed jointly in the colleges of Architecture and Medicine. A behavioral scientist, he conducts research on the effects of art and architecture on patient medical outcomes. He and his associates have researched the effects of hospital window views on recovery from surgery, the influences of abstract and representational pictures on patient outcomes in intensive care units, and how certain types of art displayed in high stress workplaces can mitigate employee anger. Among other achievements, his research is the first to document scientifically the stress reducing and health-related benefits for hospital patients of viewing nature and other attractive environments. Dr. Ulrich has developed a Theory of Psychologically Supportive Design that has become influential as a scientifically grounded but "user friendly" guide for creating successful health care facilities.

Dr. Ulrich has published many articles and his research has received international scientific recognition. He is a member of the Board of Directors of The Center for Health Design, California, and serves as cochair of its national Research Committee.

Rev. Jo Clare Wilson, a native of Nashville, Tennessee, is ordained in the Christian Church (Disciples of Christ) and has served as a pastor in Nashville, a pastoral counselor in a mental health center in rural Nebraska, and a chaplain and clinical pastoral education supervisor in Ann Arbor, Michigan.

In 1991, Rev. Wilson became coordinator of clinical pastoral education at Memorial Medical Center in Savannah, Georgia. In 1996, she began her own business, CareGivers Consultants, Inc., in which she outsourced pastoral care and education within the hospital and hospice community and, with a Robert Wood Johnson grant, worked to provide training in local congregations for AIDS Care Team members. In October 2000, Rev. Wilson began at the HealthCare Chaplaincy as director of pastoral care and education at Griffin Hospital. Her work involves providing pastoral and spiritual care for patients, families, and staff members, teaching students in the clinical pastoral education program, and working with the parish nurse and community health programs.

Introduction: The Emergence of Patient-Centered Care and the Planetree Model

Susan B. Frampton

Since the dawn of human time, providing care to the ill, distressed, and injured has been a personal calling. Individuals touched by the suffering of their fellows strove to find ways to relieve pain, provide emotional comfort, and derive spiritual meaning from the often mysterious vicissitudes of the human condition. The shamans, witches, and medicine men of our ancestors have been transformed in Western society into our present-day nurses, physicians, counselors, and chaplains. Specialization in the helping professions has grown tremendously, health care has become a trillion-dollar business in the United States alone, and patients have become health care consumers.

Consumerism is certainly not a phenomenon limited to health care; it has become a defining characteristic of our social fabric, driving our economy and fundamentally changing the way we do business. Today's consumers expect a different kind of purchasing experience from what they had in the past. Whether they are buying coffee or a car, enjoying a movie, or being cared for in a hospital, they expect options that are tailored to their needs and desires. Common in today's marketplace are myriad choices, such as six varieties of fresh-brewed coffee with eight different flavor shots, and cappuccino, mocha latte, and iced espresso in small, medium, and large sizes, decaffeinated or fat-free. Also available are mega-movieplexes with twenty screens and fifteen movie choices, with new releases showing every hour on the hour in plush stadium seating with stereo surround sound. Purchase your tickets in advance at home via the Internet, at credit card kiosks in the lobby, or in the old-fashioned way.

Successful businesses in today's consumer-driven society have done a masterful job of identifying what is important to their customers, not only about products themselves but also about the delivery of the products. It's not enough for a hotel to provide an acceptable room to a regular business traveler today. Many hotels keep that traveler's preferences in a computer file so that the customer doesn't even have to ask for the nonsmoking room at the end of a corridor on the ground floor, with Evian stocked in the minifridge when he or she checks in.

While the rest of the world has embraced the consumer revolution and has used it to improve service and build customer satisfaction and loyalty, hospitals and health care have been slow to change. We have defined our product too narrowly as a good technical or physical outcome. And while our technology may be state-of-the-art, our delivery has been pathetic. We have lost sight of the primary reason patients come to us. They come not just for medical care, nursing care, and health care; they also come to us for *caring*.

They come to us when they are most vulnerable, looking for support, comfort, and hope. They come to be heard, to be helped, and we make them wait too long in our emergency rooms, seated in uncomfortable, ugly furniture. We isolate them from their loved ones, treat them like children, and withhold information. We require our regular patients with chronic conditions to fill out the same information on the same forms, even though we have asked for this information on numerous previous occasions. We put up glass barriers in our waiting areas and nursing stations so that our patients and their families won't disturb us while we work. We spend too little time listening and answering questions, and we spend too much time on documentation and filing insurance forms.

Health care often takes the same insensitive approach to dealing with another of its most valuable resources—its employees.

Good people with caring hearts enter the health professions to serve patients. Disenchanted with an industry that often puts the bottom line before human needs, nurses in particular are burning out, and fewer young people are choosing health care professions. Coupled with an increase in the demand for health care, these forces are fueling a labor shortage that threatens to undermine health care for years to come (Advisory Board Company, 1999).

The vast majority of health care organizations have not kept pace with the consumer revolution. They continue to put technology first. They don't respect the time or the dignity of their patients. They continue to place people in flimsy, open-backed gowns and wheel them past the lobby or the cafeteria on gurneys. The patients stare up at harsh fluorescent ceiling lights on their way to a one-hour wait in radiology, where they hope they won't run into their neighbor, waiting in the same room, fully clothed, reading outdated copies of *Good Housekeeping*.

If one didn't know better, one might think that hospitals set out to design systems that provide the most sophisticated technical care but deliver the worst possible experience to sick people. This was certainly the impression of one particular patient, Angelica Thieriot, when she was hospitalized in the mid-1970s with a life-threatening condition. Thieriot experienced the classic dysfunctional dichotomy in American medicine—the separation of body from mind. The best of Western technologic medicine was made available to diagnose and treat her physical symptoms, but little attention was paid to her emotional, social, and spiritual needs. Hospital policies limited the time her family could be by her side to support her. Paternalistic attitudes on the part of providers prevented the sharing of information and explanation that would have assuaged her fears. Austere institutional surroundings did little to comfort her and only served to increase her anxiety. Eventually discharged when her symptoms resolved, Thieriot noted that spending time in a hospital was more traumatic than having a life-threatening illness.

Within a year, both her son and her father-in-law were hospitalized, and Thieriot received a "crash course" in hospitals from the family's perspective. Relegated to distant family waiting areas and being in limbo—not knowing what was happening to loved ones— she found the family experience as depersonalizing and terrifying as her own experience as a patient.

The Planetree Model

Motivated to action by these events, as well as by her vision for a more healing hospital experience for patients and families, Thieriot, in 1978, founded Planetree as a nonprofit organization. Taking its name from the sycamore, or planetree, under which Hippocrates taught his students, the organization dedicated itself to radically changing the way health care was delivered. Over the centuries, medicine had lost its holistic, patient-centered focus, and Planetree vowed to reclaim that for patients. Everything in the hospital setting was evaluated from the perspective of the patient. Every element of the organization's culture was assessed, based on whether it enhanced or detracted from personalizing, demystifying, and humanizing the patient experience. A premium was placed on making information available to health care consumers, enabling them to be informed partners in their care.

Planetree's first step was to establish a consumer health resource center, which opened in 1981 in San Francisco. The center was a place where the lay public had access to medical and health information, as well as in-depth research services. The resource center initially offered users a library of over two thousand health books and medical texts, a clipping file of current medical research, a catalogue of support groups and agencies, and a bookstore. Such a wealth of health information resources was an unheard-of luxury at a time when patients were still routinely barred from entering a hospital or medical school library.

The Planetree Health Resource Center became a national model, subsequently helping other organizations establish successful libraries throughout the country. The center developed a widely used consumer cataloging system known as the Planetree Classification Scheme, which continues to be used by health resource centers around the world.

The History of the Planetree Model

Access to health and medical information was only one aspect of Planetree's vision for personalizing health care. In June 1985, with funding from The Henry J. Kaiser Family Foundation and The San Francisco Foundation, a major milestone was reached with the opening of the Planetree model hospital unit. The first of five Planetree model hospital sites, the thirteen-bed medical-surgical unit at Pacific Presbyterian Medical Center in San Francisco, California, was like no other hospital unit in existence at that time. This unit was the culmination of years of grassroots effort to create a truly new model of care in the hospital setting. Its creation launched one of the most far-reaching experiments in the realm of consumer-responsive, patient-centered care ever attempted in this country.

Using findings from numerous focus groups with patients, families, and staff members, the innovative medical-surgical unit was designed to offer the latest medical technology in an environment that was comforting and supportive. The thirteen-bed unit was a pioneering effort to change the way patients experienced hospitals—from impersonal and intimidating institutions to nurturing, healing, and educational environments.

Over seventy physicians admitted patients to the Planetree unit. Each agreed to commit to the philosophy of patient education, participation, and family involvement. Planetree patients had the opportunity to develop direct communication with their doctors, in which they were encouraged to ask questions, request information, and participate in their care. This open communication benefited both patients and their physicians, in that the prescribed treatment plan continually reflected the patients' own goals.

An atmosphere conducive to healing was created by Planetree's original architect, Roslyn Lindheim. Lindheim, a professor at the University of California at Berkeley, had studied hospitals and therapeutic environments throughout the world and had incorporated the most significant aspects into the model unit. The result was a remarkable transformation of a typical hospital environment into a physical space that promoted healing, learning, and patient participation.

Standard partitions between patients and staff members were removed, leaving open and airy work spaces. Soothing colors were chosen, and each room was decorated differently to be as individual as the patient who occupied it. A patient lounge was created to be a comfortable place where patients, families, and friends could relax, share a meal, or watch a movie. The lounge also served as a satellite resource center providing medical and health information on the unit.

The Planetree unit included a kitchenette, where patients and family members were encouraged to prepare meals, using hospital food or food they'd brought from home. Hungry patients were never told that they would have to wait until hospital staff members delivered the next meal. The Planetree kitchenette was stocked with a variety of healthy snack foods, including fruit, yogurt, crackers, and herb teas.

Acknowledging that hospitals are often perceived as frightening, unfamiliar places, staff members encouraged the patient's family and friends to spend time there as a comfort to the patient, helping him or her avoid loneliness and isolation. Visiting hours on the Planetree unit were unrestricted, and children were permitted to visit. Family members and friends who wanted to stay overnight were accommodated either in the patient's room or on a sofa bed in the patient lounge nearby. Patients were encouraged to wear their own pajamas and display family photos on conveniently located shelves.

Families were encouraged to participate in the education, physical care, and emotional support of the patient. One specific person was designated to be a care partner, becoming more actively involved in that patient's care. The care partner was often the person who would continue to care for the patient after he or she was discharged from the hospital. The care partner worked closely with the nurses in a supportive, supervised environment to learn whatever skills might be needed—to perform tasks as simple as helping a patient bathe or dress or as complex as adjusting a portable ventilator. By helping the care partner feel comfortable in caring for the patient, the transition toward going home was often easier.

The model unit provided a wide variety of educational opportunities for patients, including written materials, audiotapes and videotapes, and personal instruction by the staff. Patients, care partners, family members, and friends were invited to make use of the educational resources.

Patients were given information packets specific to their diagnosis and needs. These packets, provided by the Planetree Health Resource Center, included basic medical information, listings of support groups, and other resources that might be helpful after the patient had gone home. In addition, information about complementary therapies, such as massage or stress management, was provided.

The Planetree philosophy stressed that one of the most valuable learning resources available was the patient's own medical chart. Patients were encouraged to read their charts daily, ask questions and discuss findings, and participate in the decisions affecting their care. Patients were also encouraged to keep written records of their experiences and observations in patient progress notes, which became a permanent part of their medical chart if they so desired.

It was the goal of the Planetree unit to help patients not only get well faster but also stay well longer, possibly avoiding future hospitalizations. With this in mind, Planetree created a self-medication program, enabling appropriate patients to administer their own medications while they are hospitalized. Patients were given fact sheets listing uses and possible side effects, and a pharmacist was available to answer questions. The patient gradually assumed more responsibility, taking the medication at the appropriate time and charting that it was taken. This learning process often avoided the problems that occurred when a patient went home with several medications and was unsure what, when, or how much should be taken.

While reducing the stress of hospitalization, the Planetree unit also educated patients about ways to reduce the stress in their daily lives. Volunteers who were specialists in relaxation, visualization, and massage offered their services at no charge, helping to make the hospital stay more relaxing and rewarding.

While drawing on the latest technology in Western medicine, the model unit also attempted to nurture the healing resources within each patient. Although medicine traditionally draws on the body's resources to heal, Planetree believes that by incorporating the mind and spirit into this process, healing can take place faster and more completely. In an effort to meet the needs of the whole person (body, mind, and spirit), the Planetree unit incorporated the arts into its healing environment.

To help meet the human need for beauty, the patient rooms were decorated with photographs of English gardens and artwork on loan from local art museums. Patients were provided with portable cassette players and offered a large selection of musical options and relaxation tapes. Comedy movies were also available, as well as a selection of books on tape.

Research on the Model Unit

The original Planetree unit was structured as a three-year demonstration project, serving as a model for hospitals and health care providers throughout the country. As part of the pilot project, the University of Washington agreed to evaluate the impact of the Planetree unit on the patient experience. The evaluation was also designed to study the level of satisfaction among nurses and doctors on the Planetree unit, its effect on the quality of patient care, and its cost-effectiveness. Significant findings, described more fully in Chapter Eleven, included increases in patient satisfaction with the environment of the unit, the technical quality of the care provided, and the education provided. Study results summarized the project as a "successful example of patient-centered hospital care" (Martin and others, 1998, p. 133).

The success of this unique experiment generated a great deal of interest. Four additional model sites were subsequently implemented between 1987 and 1990 to refine the model in diverse settings. These sites included the Samuels Planetree unit (cardiac unit) at Beth Israel Medical Center in New York City, a twenty-eight-bed medical-surgical unit at San Jose Medical Center in San Jose, California, the large subacute patient units at Delano Regional Medical Center in Delano, California, and Mid-Columbia Medical Center, a community hospital in The Dalles, Oregon—the first organization to implement Planetree concepts hospital-wide.

By the early 1990s, hundreds of tour groups from hospitals across the country and around the world had visited the model sites and worked with the Planetree organization to enhance patient care at their institutions. Managed care was rapidly expanding, hospital budgets were shrinking, the number of beds was declining, and competition for patients was growing. Executive teams were looking for innovative strategies to improve patient satisfaction and differentiate their hospitals in an increasingly competitive health care marketplace. One such team from a community hospital in Connecticut believed that the Planetree model was the right strategy for them. Pioneering a new relationship with Planetree, Griffin Hospital in Derby, Connecticut, became the first Planetree affiliate—in 1992. Given this more flexible approach to Planetree implementation, additional hospitals and health systems followed suit, forming what is now known as the Planetree Alliance of Hospitals and Healthcare Organizations. The alliance is a rapidly growing network of hospitals across the United States and Europe, pioneering innovative solutions to the changing needs of health care consumers.

Patient-Centered Care and Health Care Consumerism

The story of Planetree mirrors the journey of patient-centered care through the evolution of health care delivery during the last quarter century. From radical idealist philosophy to mainstream business differentiation strategy, patient-centered care has become a well-accepted approach to improving health care quality from the increasingly respected perspective of the patient/consumer. No longer passive recipients, today's educated consumers are a powerful force for change. They are driving a transformation in health care no less profound than that brought about by the technological breakthroughs of the twentieth century. The rapid rise in health care consumerism can be traced to several trends. The first has been the steady increase in health care costs. As these costs have risen, so, too, has the amount consumers are expected to pay out of their own pockets. Employers have shifted more and more of the burden of health care coverage onto employees. In response, individuals have increased both their knowledge and their scrutiny of how their health care dollar is being spent, and they are demanding new levels of value and service (KPMG, 1998; Press Ganey Associates, 1999; Ganey and Drain, 1998).

At the same time, we've undergone an explosion in the amount of information available in all areas—in particular, on health-related topics. The ease of access to this information, especially that provided by the Internet, has created an exceptionally well-informed population (Larkin, 1999; McLaughlin, 2001; Eng and others, 1998; Ernst & Young LLP, 1998). Combine these trends with an increasingly mobile American population, with more and more people willing to travel greater distances to get what they want, whether it is a house in the country, a job in the city, or the best patient-care experience in the region, and the result is the new health care consumerism.

What do consumers want from the health care system today? They assume that they will receive the highest-quality technical care. However, they also want respect, kindness, privacy, information, autonomy, choices, and inclusion. In addition, they expect healthy, delicious food in a homelike environment, preferably with their family, friends, and pets around them.

Although conditions have improved, hospitals have a long way to go in meeting patients' needs. Nothing less than a complete transformation of health care organizational culture is needed. At the heart of this transformation is the need to listen to what patients feel are barriers to their health and healing and to find ways of removing these barriers (American College of Healthcare Executives, 1999; Bezold, 1999; Coile, 2002).

Part One: The Nine Elements of Planetree Patient-Centered Care

Planetree embarked on this journey to identify and remove barriers with its original model site projects. Through these early initiatives, the nine elements of patient-centered care emerged, and each was adapted over time, first by the model Planetree hospitals and later by the many Planetree affiliate hospitals that followed (Frampton, 2000, 2001; Freedman, 2001). Each of these nine elements is described in the first nine chapters of the book, drawing from the experiences and insights of the organizations that have implemented them over the past two decades.

In Chapter One, Laura Gilpin explores human interactions and how they can be shaped to create an organizational culture that is truly healing and patient-centered. She presents numerous strategies employed by Planetree affiliate hospitals that have successfully cultivated the degree of understanding and ownership necessary to change employee beliefs and practices.

Candace Ford and Laura Gilpin present the Planetree model's approach to patient and family education in Chapter Two. Strategies— including development of health resource centers, customized patient information packets, bedside collaborative care conferences, patient pathways, self-medication programs, and open medical chart policies—are detailed.

In Chapter Three, Susan Edgman-Levitan discusses the strong case for involvement of the patient's social support network, as well as examples of specific policies and programs that have been implemented to achieve this involvement in health care settings around the country.

Kathy Reinke and Carol Ryczek present best practice examples of using nutrition to nurture the soul as well as the body in Chapter Four. The symbolic role of food as welcome agent and comfort is explored within the context of the hospital environment. Practical suggestions for changing the image of hospital food are offered.

Chaplains George Handzo and Jo Clare Wilson review, in Chapter Five, recent research linking spirituality and health. They provide a variety of examples of ways in which patient-centered hospitals have addressed the spiritual needs of patients, their families, and employees.

In Chapter Six, Michele Spatz and Dianne Storby explore the role of human touch, and, in particular, massage, in enhancing the experience of patients, families, and staff members. Strategies that have been used successfully for incorporating these services are presented, both for inpatient and outpatient environments.

Roger Ulrich and Laura Gilpin provide, in Chapter Seven, a comprehensive, science-grounded review of theory, research, and practice relating to how the arts (visual, musical, and theatrical) affect patient outcomes. The presentation of evidence-based guidelines for selecting health care art in particular will be extremely useful for readers.

In Chapter Eight, David Katz presents a thorough treatment of the state of integrative medicine in both inpatient and outpatient settings. Beginning with a balanced review of the pros and cons of inclusion of complementary and alternative therapies, he provides a thoughtful examination of a sometimes controversial topic. Specific models and examples from Planetree hospitals that have embraced integrative medicine are presented.

Since Planetree is well known for innovation within the realm of architecture and design, environmental elements are explored in Chapter Nine by Bruce Arneill and Karrie Frasca-Beaulieu. Practical approaches to interior and exterior renovation that support patient-centered care are presented in detail. From the use of space to the application of colors and lighting, examples of best practices are offered that stimulate thinking and challenge assumptions about what the hospital's physical environment can offer to patients.

Part Two: Future Directions for Patient-Centered Care

The core elements just presented have stood the test of time, but their expression has flourished in a thousand different ways. As employees at hospitals across the country have had the opportunity and responsibility to bring patient-centered care to life in their organizations, a limitless well of creativity has been tapped. Some of their best ideas are presented in the case examples included throughout Chapters One through Nine, where the core elements are presented in depth. These ideas took initial root primarily in acute care hospitals, but in many cases they have been adapted to outpatient and subacute care settings, as patient care has continued to shift to these settings.

Chapters Ten through Sixteen build on the present foundations of patient-centered care, and then they take them a step further. What will the truly healing hospital of the future be like? What impact will it have on larger issues in the communities it serves? Is it economical to deliver this kind of care? What impact does it have on staff recruitment and retention? How do you acquire the support and participation of the medical staff? What role will hospitals play in the continuing evolution of the holistic care of their patients' mind, body, and spirit? These issues will be explored in the context of transforming the culture of health care as we know it.

In Chapter Ten, Patrick Charmel presents the business case for patient-centered care. Drawing from case examples of hospitals that have seen impressive increases in patient and employee satisfaction levels, patient volume increases, and decreases in malpractice claims, he makes the case for "doing well by doing good."

Steven Horowitz echoes these sentiments in Chapter Eleven, exploring particular benefits to the medical staff of participating in a patient-centered model. Effective strategies for gaining physician support are discussed.

Chapter Twelve presents a wealth of ideas for improving nursing staff recruitment and retention. Charlene Honeycutt and Phyllis Stoneburner review present challenges and opportunities of the current and growing health care workforce shortages.

In Chapter Fourteen, Allan Komarek translates the Planetree model from acute to subacute and long-term care settings. How do we create the ideal nursing home setting? What could patient-centered care look like to frail elderly rehab patients or the comatose trauma victim during extended hospital stays?

Chapters Thirteen and Fifteen take us into the not-so-distant future. Trevor Hancock presents the latest information from the "green" hospitals movement thriving in Canada and Europe and its early advances in the United States. Leland Kaiser takes us onto the spiritual frontier in health care, envisioning a bold new path to true mind-body-spirit health care.

Finally, in Chapter Sixteen, Randall Carter and the editors summarize the challenges and opportunities for further development of patient-centered care in healing health care environments. Looking at today's best practices in combination with emerging trends in health care, they suggest where we should focus our attention in order to meet and exceed the needs and desires of our patients, their families, and our staff.

Derby, Connecticut   Susan B. Frampton
February 2003

References

Advisory Board Company. *Nursing Executive Center National RN Survey.* Washington, D.C.: Advisory Board Company, 1999.

American College of Healthcare Executives. *Patient- and Family-Centered Care: Good Values, Good Business.* Conference Brochure. Miami Beach, Fla.: American College of Healthcare Executives, Mar. 22–23, 1999.

Bezold, C. "Health Care Faces a Dose of Change." *The Futurist,* Apr. 1999, pp. 30–34.

Coile, R., Jr., and Russell, C. *FUTURESCAN 2002, A Forecast of Healthcare Trends 2002–2006.* Chicago: Health Administration Press, American College of Healthcare Executives, 2002.

Eng, T. R., and others. "Access to Health Information and Support: A Public Highway or a Private Road?" *JAMA,* 1998, *280*(15), 1371–1375.

Ernst & Young LLP. "Built to Last Means Built to Change." *Medicare+Choice and The New Health Care Consumerism.* June 1998.

Frampton, S. "Planetree Patient-Centered Care and the Healing Arts." *Complementary Health Practice Review,* 2000, *7*(1), 17–19.

Frampton, S. "Vantage Point: The Planetree Model." In N. Faass (ed.), *Integrating Complementary Medicine into Health Systems.* Gaithersburg, Md.: Aspen, 2001.

Freedman, D. H. "Redesigning the Hospital Environment." In N. Faass (ed.), *Integrating Complementary Medicine into Health Systems.* Gaithersburg, Md.: Aspen, 2001.

Ganey, R., and Drain, M. "Patient Satisfaction: What You See Is What You Get." *Trustee,* Nov./Dec. 1998, pp. 6–10.

KPMG. "Consumerism in Health Care: New Voices." *Consumerism in Health Care Research Study Findings.* Jan. 1998, pp. 6–24.

Larkin, H. "Programs to Boost Patient Satisfaction Payoff in Many Ways, CEO's Say." *AHA News,* June 21, 1999, p. 1.

Martin, D., and others. "Randomized Trial of a Patient-Centered Hospital Unit." *Patient Education and Counseling,* 1998, (34), pp. 125–133.

McLaughlin, N. "Great Expectations: Providers Better Pay Attention to Educated Patients." *Modern Healthcare,* Feb. 26, 2001, p. 24.

Press Ganey Associates. "One Million Patients Have Spoken: Who Will Listen?" *The Satisfaction Monitor,* 1999.

Putting Patients First

Part One

Nine Elements of Patient-Centered Care

1

The Importance of Human Interaction

Laura Gilpin

When Angelica Thieriot, the founder of Planetree, was faced with an acute illness she felt it was more frightening to be hospitalized than to face a life-threatening health crisis. "First do no harm" is the golden rule of health care. Yet many patients leave hospitals, as Thieriot did, feeling abused, traumatized, and dehumanized. In an attempt to alleviate physical suffering, hospitals seem to create, or at least exacerbate, emotional suffering. Planetree's goal has always been to change the way patients experience hospitals and other health care settings.

Roslyn Lindheim, professor of architecture at the University of California at Berkeley, became one of Planetree's founding board members. She had traveled extensively and studied for many years—in a variety of cultures—why people get sick and, more important, what keeps them well and helps them heal. What she found corroborated Thieriot's own personal experiences: that patients want and need supportive human relationships, a sense that they are valued and respected, a sense of control over their lives, and an opportunity for meaningful participation (Lindheim and Syme, 1983; Lindheim, 1979, 1981, 1985). These became the foundations of the Planetree model.

As Planetree began to expand the model beyond the initial model hospital unit, which opened in San Francisco in 1985, the components that had been put into operation on the first unit were examined for their relevance to patients in other environments and geographic locations. Planetree felt that the best way to obtain this information was to go directly to patients to ask them about their perceptions. Over the next decade, the Planetree staff conducted numerous focus groups with hospitalized patients and those who had been recently discharged. The information gathered in these focus groups was later supported by similar findings from focus groups and an extensive survey conducted by the Picker Institute in Boston (Gerteis, Edgman-Levitan, Daley, and Delbanco, 1993).

Many of the aspects that patients focus on have little to do with the quality of their medical care and far more to do with the quality of how their medical care is delivered. When Press Ganey Associates (1999) studied 139,830 former patients from 225 hospitals, it found that none of the top fifteen factors determining patient satisfaction related to whether the patient's health improved while in the hospital. Instead, many of the factors that most highly correlate with patient satisfaction refer to interactions with hospital staff.

While the health care system excels at measuring and improving the *what* and *why* of medical care, patients themselves are more concerned with the *how* and *by whom*. In a technological era that values the objectivity of science, little regard has been given to the subjective experience of patients. Subjectivity is often relegated to the realm of "patient satisfaction" and referred to as "soft science." Although patient satisfaction is viewed as vital to the hospital's financial health, it is rarely perceived as having an effect on the health outcomes of those who receive care. New medications, procedures, and other advances in medical care are often studied extensively, whereas the manner in which these advances are delivered is intentionally factored out. As Leland Kaiser points out, "If it doesn't matter how the care is delivered, why do pharmaceutical companies conduct double-blind studies?" (personal interview, Apr. 11, 2001).

What underlies many of the issues raised in focus groups and patient satisfaction surveys is an area that medical science finds difficult to define, much less to quantify. It involves the vague and illusive but vital area of human interactions. How do we communicate caring? How do we ensure that patients feel respected? How do we encourage patients to ask questions? How do we honor patients' dignity when dignity may be defined differently by each patient?

When a nurse or other caregiver enters a patient's room to give a medication, deliver a meal, or complete any task, what really takes place? Medical science would have us believe that completing the task alone is enough. Quality is seen as a measure of how skillfully and efficiently each task is performed. But from the patient's perspective, every task is more than the delivery of medical services. It is an opportunity for human interaction. Planetree has always believed that how care is delivered is as important as the care itself.

The Role of Human Interactions in Health and Healing

Positive interactions between patients and staff members are obviously important from the perspective of patient satisfaction, but do they contribute to health and healing? Being nice to patients may be good business, but is it good medicine? While few studies have been done in a hospital setting examining the health benefits of interactions with staff members, there are many other examples suggesting that social connections have a positive effect on health outcomes.

In a seventeen-year follow-up on the 6,848 adults who participated in an Alameda County study, it was found that women who were socially isolated were found to have a significantly elevated risk of dying of cancer of all sites and men with few social connections also showed significantly poorer cancer survival rates (Reynolds and Kaplan, 1990). David Spiegel, in his book *Living Beyond Limits* (1993), cites many studies linking cancer survival to social support. Spiegel proposes several possibilities for the positive effects, including the notion that social support may affect the quality of a patient's basic activities, such as eating and sleeping, and may help patients interact more effectively with their physicians.

He also suggests that social support may serve as a buffer against stress, possibly decreasing the production of stress hormones such as cortisol and prolactin. Stress is known to have a deleterious effect on the immune system Heart disease, the leading cause of death in the United States, has also been closely correlated with a low level of social support. At Duke University, a study of nearly fourteen hundred men and women diagnosed with coronary artery disease found that 50 percent of those who were socially isolated died within five years, compared with 17 percent of those living with a spouse (Williams and others, 1992). Many other studies report findings that loneliness, isolation, and lack of social support contribute to illness and premature death (Blazer, 1982; Berkman, Leo-Summers, and Horwitz, 1992; Wiklund and others, 1988). Dean Ornish, in his book *Love and Survival* (1988), cites many studies supporting the link between social connectedness and health outcomes.

Social support also seems to alleviate the physiological effects of stress. Kamarck, Manuck, and Jennings (1990) found that when women were asked to complete a mental math problem alone, their systolic blood pressure and heart rate were significantly higher than if they were allowed to have a friend with them. In a similar study, participants were asked to give a speech, either alone, in the presence of a supportive person, or in the presence of a nonsupportive person. Those with a supportive person present during the speech experienced the least change in blood pressure, whereas those in the presence of a nonsupportive person exhibited the greatest rise in blood pressure—even more than those who gave the speech alone (Lepore, Mata Allen, and Evans, 1993).

Several of the studies previously cited define social connectedness as being married, having a confidant, meeting with others in ongoing support groups, or participating in other activities that could foster and maintain long-term relationships. (The importance of these relationships will be covered in depth in Chapter Three, which discusses the role of family and friends.) One could make the case that a brief interaction with a nurse, laboratory technician, or other health care provider might not be enduring or significant enough to have any effect on the patient. But the Lepore study suggests that positive support during stressful events can minimize stress, whereas a nonsupportive person can exacerbate the stress. The stress of giving a speech might be comparable to what patients experience when undergoing a frightening medical procedure.

It is not uncommon in focus groups to hear descriptions from patients of how one caring person, even one brief interaction with a caring person—someone who listened to or supported the patient at a difficult time—changed the patient's experience. Not infrequently, patients state that the person who listened or seemed most caring was a hospital housekeeper. This is one reason why Planetree considers everyone who works in a hospital or in any related health care field to be a caregiver. From a patient's perspective, the title or job description of someone caring is of less importance than the fact that the caregiver is providing emotional support.

It is hoped that in the future more studies will examine the role of short-term interactions on health outcomes in a hospital setting. Does pain medication work more effectively if administered by someone who seems to care if the pain is alleviated? Does kindness reduce the level of stress hormones in patients? Do patients sleep better without the use of sedatives or heal faster from surgery in an environment where supportive interactions with staff members are common?

The Role of Human Interactions in Patient Satisfaction

Until we have answers to questions regarding the potential health benefits of human interactions, we can rely only on the fact that these interactions figure prominently in measures of patient satisfaction. Many questions asked on a typical patient satisfaction survey solicit the patient's perceptions about the manner in which care was delivered. How friendly and courteous was the staff in various departments? How caring were the nurses? How willing were nurses to answer questions? How well were family members kept informed? Rarely are questions asked about the medical care itself. Was the surgical procedure performed correctly? Did you receive the correct medications? Were falls prevented? The quality of the medical care itself is usually tracked through incident reports, performance improvement measures, and reviews of adverse patient outcomes. Patient satisfaction, while not considered "hard science," is currently the best measure of the effects of human interactions on the patient's overall hospital experience.

The first study of patient satisfaction at a Planetree site was conducted by the University of Washington at the initial Planetree model unit. In this randomized, controlled trial of 618 patients hospitalized between 1986 and 1990, patient outcomes on the Planetree unit were compared with those on other medical-surgical units. Planetree patients were found to be significantly more satisfied with their hospital stay, their nursing care, the social support they received, the environment on the unit, and the education they were given. Planetree patients reported more involvement in their care during their hospitalization. While there were few differences in health behaviors between Planetree patients and those in the control group, Planetree patients reported better mental health status and role functioning initially after discharge. Costs were found to be the same (Martin and others, 1998).

Other Planetree sites have also measured patient satisfaction by using a variety of instruments, including Press Ganey, Picker, and Planetree surveys. Saint Joseph Community Hospital in Mishawaka, Indiana, found that its patient satisfaction increased in each of seven quarters, representing an 8 percent increase during the two years it conducted Planetree staff retreats, training 80 percent of the staff. Beth Israel Medical Center in New York City found that patient satisfaction increased on the Samuels Planetree unit over the two years following initial implementation. The unit was initially ranked seventeenth out of eighteen clinical units in patient satisfaction and became one of the top two in approximately one year. Griffin Hospital in Derby, Connecticut, found that patient satisfaction increased from 83 to 97 percent during the four-year period in which it fully implemented the Planetree model throughout the hospital. Hospital inpatient volume increased by 27.5 percent between 1999 and 2002, compared with a 7.7 percent statewide average increase. Staff-to-patient ratios remained the same, and operating expense per discharge declined.

There is a misconception that supportive interactions require more staff or more time and are therefore more costly. Although labor costs are a substantial part of any hospital budget, the interactions themselves add nothing to the budget. Kindness is free. Listening to patients or answering their questions costs nothing. It could be argued that negative interactions—alienating patients, being unresponsive to their needs, or limiting their sense of control—can be very costly in lost patient revenues and perhaps litigation. Angry, frustrated, or frightened patients may be combative, withdrawn, and less cooperative, requiring far more time than it would have taken to interact with them initially in a positive way.

Putting Concepts into Action

Achieving high patient satisfaction is likely the goal of every hospital. Mission statements from hospitals large and small, urban and rural, for-profit and not-for-profit, usually include words such as "caring," "compassionate," "respect," and "dignity"—all of which reflect the quality of human interactions. But putting these concepts into practice can be a difficult task. Providing patients with what they want—being valued and respected, having a sense of control, and being provided with opportunities to participate—cannot be achieved solely by implementing programs or policies. Care-partner programs, unlimited visiting hours, and open-chart policies are of little use if they are implemented in an environment that has not addressed the quality of fundamental human interactions.

Personalized Care

Planetree has focused extensively on working with hospital staff members by conducting retreats for all hospital employees, to encourage supportive interactions with each patient. Some hospitals have tried to identify and define specific behaviors or interactions that are perceived to be beneficial, but many Planetree sites focus on the concept of providing each patient with personalized care. Personalized care is a vital concept that needs to be reinforced with the hospital staff, and each patient is a unique individual with different likes and needs. What is appropriate for one patient may be inappropriate for another. One patient may wake up at 5 A.M., ready for a bath and breakfast, whereas another patient may routinely stay awake until 3 A.M. and wish to sleep until noon. Positive interactions require personalizing the care.

Although most staff members endorse the concept of personalization, change is difficult. Standardization rather than personalization has been the rule throughout health care for many decades. Even if there are no written policies, many unwritten perceptions form the dominant organizational culture at many institutions. Patients are weighed at 5 A.M. Bed baths are given in the morning. Blood products are usually administered at night. There is typically no medical reason for the timing of these standard hospital procedures. Patients who wish to sleep late can be weighed at the same time each evening so that the information is available when the physicians make rounds in the morning. Bed baths can be given in the evening. Blood products can be administered during the day so that the patient's sleep is not disturbed by frequent checks of vital signs. Common sense is often overridden by corporate culture. "That's not the way we do things here" and "we've never done it that way before" are frequent refrains when efforts are made to implement change. Organizational transformation helps staff members question every hospital routine, even those held most sacred, so that personalization becomes standard.

Presence

The most important human interactions are the ones that are appropriate and wanted by the patient. But personalization requires that staff members be "present." Someone has to notice the patient and acknowledge and get to know that unique individual. Every task, whether changing a dressing or sweeping the floor, provides staff members with the opportunity to interact with and get to know the patient. One patient revealed to a housekeeper that he was terrified about his surgery the next day because his brother had died a few years earlier during the same operation. This interaction provided information that enabled the surgeon to talk with the patient about his concerns. In some hospitals, the housekeeper would have been reprimanded for "wasting time" by visiting with a patient.

Nurses and other clinical caregivers are often trained to be "professional." This term is frequently thought of as meaning objective, emotionally detached, or distant. Introductions in Planetree staff retreats focus on "Who are you really?" We believe that if each employee feels accepted as a unique individual, he or she is more likely to appreciate the uniqueness of each patient he or she comes into contact with. Some Planetree hospitals use terms such as "authenticity" and "being there." If a caregiver says the right words and performs the right actions but isn't paying attention to the patient, the implication to the patient is that he or she is nothing more than a set of tasks to be accomplished. Being present enables caregivers to get to know the patient so that the care can be personalized.

Patient Advocacy

Another important aspect of personalized care is patient advocacy: What do we do with the information obtained regarding what the patient wants? Who will support patients in obtaining what they perceive they need? Who will be the patient's advocate?

Nurses frequently fill the role of patient advocate but often at a significant price. "Going to bat" for a patient sometimes means challenging the health care system or breaking established rules. In many hospitals, this puts the nurse in an awkward situation. Being a "good" caregiver from the patient's perspective may mean being a troublesome employee from management's perspective. In an organization that supports personalization and patient advocacy, nurses and other caregivers no longer have to bend or break rules to support the needs of patients.

At one Planetree site, an acutely ill patient requested to go to a family reunion in another state. He felt that because of his prognosis, he would never have another opportunity to visit with his entire family. Despite his unstable condition, the patient threatened to leave the hospital against medical advice to attend the event. Rather than argue with him, the nurses and his physician worked together to make the necessary arrangements for the patient to travel. The physician contacted a physician at the other location so that the appropriate care could be provided if needed. Nurses arranged for portable oxygen and worked with the family to provide for his needs. The patient attended the reunion with no ill effects. He returned to the hospital, grateful and happy. He was eventually well enough to be discharged but died of his illness several months later.

Some staff members might not have gone to these lengths to enable a patient to attend a family event. Some might have simply let him leave on his own because it seemed easier or more expedient. There are policies for patients signing out of the hospital against medical advice but there are no policies for helping a patient travel to a family reunion. Personalized care requires advocacy and, often, creativity. No one required that the nurses take these actions. They did so because it gave them satisfaction. One of the nurses recounted this story months later, when asked to describe a time when she knew she had made a difference in someone's life.

The power of patient advocacy cannot be underestimated. When patients feel that they have an advocate, they know that they are heard, acknowledged, and understood. Their choices are being respected, which enhances their sense of control and involvement.

What Caregivers Want

Many hospitals regard employees primarily as a budgetary expense to be controlled, managed, and reduced. Although staff wages and benefits add significantly to any hospital budget, it is vital to count caregivers as assets in helping to enhance the hospital's ability to provide quality care.

Many hospitals monitor patient satisfaction every month, but staff satisfaction may only be measured every few years, if at all. Planetree was created to address how patients experience health care, but it became immediately clear that patient satisfaction and staff satisfaction go hand in hand. One cannot ask caregivers to be kind, caring, and responsive to patients if they are not being treated with the same level of kindness and consideration.

A recent survey conducted by Press Ganey Associates (1999) in eighteen hospitals found an extremely high correlation between employee and patient satisfaction. Although Planetree is often referred to as "patient-centered," it is equally focused on the nurturing of caregivers. Planetree is about human beings caring for other human beings.

Many nurses (who represent approximately 70 percent of the employees in most hospitals), as well as other staff members, choose to work in health care for the opportunity it affords to make a difference in people's lives. In years of conducting retreats and focus groups with a wide variety of caregivers at many hospitals, no one has ever stated that he or she chose to work in health care to be rude, disrespectful, and abusive to patients. Yet, at many hospitals, this is how patients describe their care. What happens to caring people who have chosen caregiving as a career, so that patients no longer perceive them as caring? How has the system made it difficult to give the kind of care that attracted many caregivers into the health care field in the first place?

Fortunately, Planetree has found that most caregivers want to give the kind of care that patients want to receive. At Griffin Hospital, 75 percent of the new clinical staff members cite the hospital's model of care (Planetree) as their reason for choosing to work at Griffin. This hospital, a Planetree affiliate for over a decade, has found that creating an environment that is better for patients (as measured by its 97 percent patient satisfaction rating) is also better for the staff. *Fortune* magazine has rated them for four consecutive years (2000, 2001, 2002, 2003) as one of the "100 Best Places to Work" in America. If a hospital is a good place to work, it is probably also a good place to be a patient.

Another reason that staff satisfaction is vital is that hospitals are now competing not only for patients but for staff members as well. According to figures from the U.S. Department of Health and Human Services, the current nursing shortage is estimated to become a national crisis by 2010. And it is not only nurses who are in short supply. Many regions of the United States are also in need of pharmacists, physical therapists, and radiology and ultrasound technologists. As a result, staff satisfaction is now receiving the attention it has always been due but rarely received.

The importance of retaining and recruiting highly qualified staff members cannot be overstated. The economic impact alone can be staggering, given that the estimated cost of recruiting, hiring, and training one nurse is up to $64,000 (Advisory Board Company, 1999). In the United States, the nursing turnover rate is approximately 20 percent, and in some regions, it is up to 35 percent (Advisory Board Company, 1999). But the human cost may be even higher as the baby boomers age and find that hospitals are unable to care for them without adequate staff. State-of-the-art medicine is nothing in the absence of qualified people to deliver the care.

But what do staff members want? Nursing salaries have been increasing over the past several years as the shortage has received widespread national attention. One might think that the problem has been solved. But while fair compensation is vital, money alone is not the answer.

The Role of Human Interactions in Staff Satisfaction

A classic study by Kenneth Kovach (1987) compared what managers perceived were the ten primary elements of staff satisfaction with what the staff members themselves ranked as important. Managers believed that the top three items that contribute to employee satisfaction are good wages, job security, and promotion/growth in the company. The employees ranked their top three as having interesting work, having appreciation of work done, and feeling "in" on things. What is perhaps most surprising is that the same factors listed by staff members as contributing most highly to their job satisfaction were ranked by managers as far less important: fifth, eighth, and tenth, respectively. What staff members want and what managers think they want are clearly at odds.

Good wages and job security are, at least in part, dependent on reimbursement rates, global economics, demographics, and other external factors. Opportunities for growth and promotion may also be linked to economic realities. Yet what matters most to employees has less to do with economics. Feeling stimulated by their work, having access to pertinent information, and feeling appreciated add little or nothing to a hospital budget. In this study, the three most important factors relating to staff satisfaction reflect the importance of human interactions.

Robert Levering (2001), consultant coordinator for *Fortune's* "100 Best Places to Work" list, states, "A great place to work is one where you trust the people you work for, have pride in what you do and enjoy the people you work with." Of the fifty-five questions on their survey, the five most highly correlated to the "100 Best" selected include

- Believability ("I can ask any reasonable question and get a straight answer.")

- Appreciation ("Management shows appreciation for good work and extra effort.")

- Collaboration ("Management genuinely seeks and responds to suggestions and ideas.")

- Sincerity ("Management shows a sincere interest in me as a person.")

- Camaraderie ("This is a fun place to work." According to Levering, this question is most highly correlated to productivity.)

All of these key elements relate to relationships and human interactions. None of them relates to wages, benefits, job security, or opportunities for promotion. Griffin's employees are not the highest paid among all hospital employees in the area, and neither are they the lowest paid. Although fair compensation is essential, financial remuneration is not enough.

The Gallup Organization has interviewed over a million employees in the past twenty-five years, and its findings are similar. Results are reported by Marcus Buckingham and Curt Coffman in their book *First Break All the Rules* (1999). They found that the "strength" of an organization could be measured by how its staff responded to twelve questions that reflect the core elements needed to "attract, focus and keep the most talented employees" (p. 28). Many of these twelve questions relate to human interactions, including:

- In the last seven days, have I received recognition or praise for doing good work?

- Does my supervisor, or someone at work, seem to care about me as a person?

- At work, do my opinions seem to count?

None of the twelve questions relates to wages, benefits, or job security.

Because of the importance of human interactions in maintaining staff satisfaction, Planetree affiliates have developed a number of ways of focusing on these issues.

Appreciation and Recognition

Many books have been written about the need to develop reward and recognition programs to acknowledge good work by staff members. Many hospitals have implemented employee of the month programs and annual awards or bonuses. Although all of these have their merit, they may fail to address the underlying culture that in many typical hospitals is focused more on punitive measures than on staff acknowledgment and recognition. In focus groups with the staff, it is not uncommon to hear that reprimands from managers and coworkers are frequent events but that appreciation is shown only once a month, at official ceremonies. Managers in focus groups express concern that by showing appreciation too often, staff members will feel that the statements are meaningless. Some managers feel that it is inappropriate to thank an employee who is simply doing his or her job.

Organizational transformation, though not a "quick fix," can profoundly change a hierarchical, punitive culture into one with an "attitude of gratitude." Reward and recognition programs are vital as formal, organizational expressions of appreciation, but they are most effective when integrated into a culture in which the appreciation and acknowledgment of others is expressed freely and frequently.

The terms most often used—*reward, recognition,* and *award*—have subtle implications that they originated in a hierarchical environment. Rewards come from the top down. Managers *recognize* worthy staff members. As hospitals become less hierarchical, such terms as *gratitude, appreciation,* and *acknowledgment* will become more common. Small gestures of appreciation, such as simply saying "thank you" more often, can become part of a new less hierarchical culture.

Whereas it is vital that managers and administrators acknowledge employees who best embody the organizational values, it is equally important that coworkers acknowledge each other and that all staff members feel comfortable expressing gratitude to anyone. Departments can thank other departments via notes, gifts, or celebrations. Staff members can express their appreciation not only to coworkers but also to managers, administrators, and physicians. To be effective, this culture change needs to be role-modeled first by every administrator, manager, and supervisor so that it becomes second nature to all employees.

At Louise Obici Memorial Hospital in Suffolk, Virginia, one of the Planetree initiative teams created a "thank-you" tree, encouraging staff members to recognize and acknowledge the good works of fellow employees. The tree, originally consisting of only a trunk and branches, was mounted on the wall of a well-traveled hallway. Employees were asked to thank their coworkers by anonymously writing their appreciation on "leaves," which were then attached to the branches. Those who were honored on the tree also received gold leaf pins. As the number of leaves increased and the tree grew, employees found it easier to value the contributions of their coworkers.

Celebrations of organizational successes, even of small accomplishments, provide wonderful opportunities to recognize the essential role that staff members play in helping the organization succeed. Whenever the hospital or individual departments achieve goals, reach desired benchmarks, or receive media attention, opportunities can be created to honor staff members for their accomplishments. They are not merely doing their jobs; they are doing their jobs exceptionally well. When New Jersey's Hackensack University Medical Center was awarded the Governor's Gold Award, festive celebrations, with music, balloons, and confetti, were held on all three shifts. The executive team and board members thanked all the employees for their contributions to making the award possible.

At Banner Health System's Thunderbird Samaritan Medical Center in Glendale, Arizona, the director of spiritual care, S. S. Sat Kartar Khalsa-Ramey, developed a Blessing of the Hands program that was initially used during Nurses' Week to acknowledge the vital work of these caregivers. The program was so well received by the nurses that it has been expanded to bless the hands of all hospital employees, to recognize the valuable work that each one of them is doing. This program has now been adapted and implemented by many Planetree hospitals and has been used successfully in a variety of settings.

Massage for the staff is another way that hospitals can express appreciation for the efforts of their caregivers. At several Planetree hospitals, a massage therapist brings a massage chair to a staff lounge so that caregivers can relax and feel nurtured during a break. Some hospitals provide gift certificates to staff members for massages as thank-you gifts to recognize their contribution to the hospital.

These simple human interactions can provide an environment of gratitude in which staff members are frequently reminded that they are valued and that their work is appreciated.

Communication and Participation

Two-way communication (being informed and being heard) is another interaction that contributes to staff satisfaction. When staff members are informed, they are better able to participate in creating a work environment in which they can thrive. However a structure needs to be established that solicits their input and encourages their ideas and solutions.

Lack of information leads to rumors and speculation. At focus groups, some employees have complained that their only source of information about the hospital comes from the local newspaper. In the old hierarchical model, staff members were kept uninformed because of the misconception that they didn't need to know, wouldn't be able to understand the information, or might be needlessly upset, particularly if the hospital was experiencing financial difficulties. In reality, staff members are usually quick to perceive problems and are fearful and frustrated when uninformed. Withholding information, or, more frequently, not making the effort to provide it, creates anxiety, mistrust, and an us versus them environment.

Employee newsletters, e-mail, written communications, and frequent town-hall-style meetings are useful tools in keeping hospital staff informed. Expecting information to pass unimpeded through several levels and still reach the staff is wishful (and hierarchical) thinking. It is not uncommon for administrators to provide information to managers who are, in turn, expected to pass the information along to the staff. Some managers are effective at relaying the information but many are not. Direct communication is the most reliable. It is also helpful for managers to understand the importance of conveying information.

In fall 2001, when a patient suspected of having inhalation anthrax was admitted to Griffin Hospital, the CEO, Patrick Charmel, informed all hospital employees as soon as the diagnosis was confirmed. The information was conveyed by using a variety of vehicles, including the hospital's intranet, one-to-one communication by the managers, and town-hall meetings open to all staff members. Rather than alarming employees, being informed created a sense of trust that proved vital, once the incident became national news.

To be most effective, communication needs to be two-way; staff members want to be kept informed, but they also need an opportunity to be heard. Having a voice in how care is delivered, and having opportunities to participate, creates an environment in which staff members can be the exceptional caregivers they want to be. It's a misconception that the benefit of staff input is simply to win their support and buy-in. The opinions, ideas, suggestions, and creative solutions of caregivers are tremendous assets in creating a healing environment for patients and an optimum working environment for the staff.

Although Planetree implementation varies at each site, a structure is established to elicit input and ideas from the staff. When Bergan Mercy Medical Center in Omaha, Nebraska, part of Alegent Health System, became a Planetree affiliate in 1993, the hospital wanted to focus first on the emergency department because of the high number of patient complaints that the department received. Initially, the staff was skeptical about the opportunity to be involved.

As Planetree implementation moved forward, caregivers began attending annual staff retreats to help keep the focus on the patient's perspective. The initial departmental team consisted of a small group of committed staff members. The team's first request was for glider-type rocking chairs for the exam rooms. Some managers expressed dismay that the initial ideas did not address the numerous patient complaints the department was receiving. Most complaints involved poor staff attitudes, long waiting times, and lack of information. But the hospital adopted a "say yes to everything" management style, so approval was given to purchase the rocking chairs. Kevin Schwedhelm, director of emergency services, describes the process of staff participation as "a snowball." Once skeptical staff members were caught up in the excitement and enthusiasm, a cascade of other valuable suggestions followed. Each decision focused not only on how the change would affect the patient's care but also on how it would affect the patient's experience of the care. The rocking chairs not only helped win staff support, they also proved to be a valuable resource in calming agitated patients.

Bergan Mercy's emergency department, rather than receiving numerous complaints, is now ranked in the 90th percentile nationwide in patient satisfaction, and its clinical outcomes are among the highest in the nation among comparable hospitals. Of the thirty-five thousand visits per year, its "walk-out" rate of patients leaving without being seen is one-half of 1 percent, whereas the national average is close to 10 percent. These achievements could not be accomplished without staff commitment.

Caregivers have valuable contributions to make toward improving the quality of care. Most caregivers want to be exceptional caregivers and know what they need to be most effective. Good leadership is vital in creating an environment that supports staff participation.

Kindness

Perhaps the simplest and most profound of all human interactions is kindness. While everyone seems to know what it is, few can define it. It goes beyond common courtesy and seems more tangible than "caring." Genuine kindness seems to bring pleasure to both the giver and the receiver. And it is often a simple place to start: How can I be kind to those around me?

But if it is so simple, it is surprising how frequently it is absent from our health care environments. The concerns that staff members in focus groups and retreats have are expressed in such questions as, How can I be kind to others when no one is kind to me? One caregiver complained that she had worked in the same hospital for years, had walked past one of the administrators on many mornings, and had never received a smile or a greeting. Many staff members comment on verbal "abuse" by physicians, managers, and coworkers.

To create a kind and caring environment for patients, we must also create a similar environment for staff members. But creating a culture of kindness cannot be mandated. Questions such as, Does someone seem to care about me as a person? reflect aspects of kindness toward caregivers that cannot be remedied by implementing programs or by writing policies or procedures.

Planetree hospitals have found a variety of ways to create a culture in which all people—patients, family members, and staff members—feel nurtured and supported. The food service department at Saint Joseph Community Hospital in Mishawaka, Indiana, found a creative way to nurture the staff in many departments. It purchased an old-fashioned wheeled coffee cart that can be taken to any department that may need extra support and nurturing. If there has been a crisis on the intensive care unit, a code in the emergency department, or a sick call in admitting, the "Planetree cart" arrives with coffee, muffins, and moral support.

The linen department at Shawano Medical Center in Shawano, Wisconsin, helps hospital employees remove stains from lab coats and uniforms. They pride themselves on being stain experts and offer their expertise to others. At Warren Memorial Hospital in Front Royal, Virginia, members of the executive team, including the CEO, work side-by-side with staff members to help out on busy days.

Kindness does not have to cost more and does not require more staff. It can be as simple as a smile, a greeting, or offering to help someone having a difficult day. When staff members feel nurtured, they are better able to care for patients. Humans are social beings, and positive interactions are vital to health.

Transforming the Organization to Support Human Interactions

Transforming a hospital or other health care organization so that it supports positive human interactions is surprisingly difficult. There is nothing complex about caring, but our health care institutions have evolved out of a paradigm that places a greater value on technology and scientific advancements than on human interactions. The very simplicity of human caring seems to create the greatest challenge in integrating it into our medical institutions. If organizational *transformation* could be accomplished through organizational *transplantation*, and if it involved the sophisticated scientific equipment of technologies, it is likely that most hospitals would be as successful at human caring as they are at delivering the modern marvels of today's medicine. But transformation often seems as illusive and difficult to define as human interactions themselves.

At many organizations, attempts at transformation stem from management initiatives with little or no involvement from the staff.

Transformation is rarely successful if it is imposed or mandated. Planetree has found that it occurs more quickly and easily, and with more lasting results, if staff members are involved in both the planning and the implementation. But many employees feel little control over the health care environment they work in. It is not uncommon for staff members to perceive an us versus them relationship with management. The first step in transformation is for the staff to realize that they *are* the organization. Change in the organizational culture can only occur when staff members are empowered and become instrumental in the process of transformation.

Over the years, Planetree has developed several ways to empower hospital staff. One is through the Planetree staff retreat, a one- or two-day training program offered at Planetree hospitals to every employee. Equally important is to establish an ongoing structure for the staff to have input into the decisions regarding the delivery of patient care. This provides an opportunity for the staff to change the rules that make it difficult to be a good caregiver or that impede positive interactions with patients or with each other.

The first Planetree staff retreat was held in January 1985. Over the past eighteen years, the retreat format and agenda have been refined. Each hospital adapts the format to best meet the needs of its staff and its organizational culture. The retreat includes experiential exercises and discussions to focus on the patient's perspective and the vital role the staff plays in personalizing the patient's care. One of the key components addressed is communication between all caregivers. Management retreats are useful in that they help support the role of the staff in implementing change.

The structure for implementing change has evolved and grown as numerous Planetree hospitals have found ways of including staff members in the decision-making process. A steering committee with ad hoc work teams has been successful at many sites. Unit- or department-based committees provide a forum for staff input regarding changes specific to each area.

The hospital's leadership also plays a key role in supporting the transformation of the organization. One of the central roles of leadership is to support and articulate the highest vision of the organization. Focusing on financial success is essential, but if that is the ultimate vision of the organization, it may be difficult to enlist staff members to achieve that goal. Most caregivers did not choose their jobs or professions with the goal of helping an institution's bottom line. Nor do patients choose to come to a hospital for the purpose of enhancing its financial viability. Organizational transformation is only possible when everyone who is part of that organization has a clear vision of the ultimate goal. For the vision to become a reality, staff members must feel valued themselves so that they can communicate a sense of caring to patients.

References

Advisory Board Company. *Nursing Executive Center National RN Survey*. Washington, D.C.: Advisory Board Company, 1999.

Berkman, L., Leo-Summers, L., and Horwitz, R. "Emotional Support and Survival After Myocardial Infarction: A Prospective, Population-Based Study of the Elderly." *Annals of Internal Medicine*, 1992, *117*(12), 1003–1009.

Blazer, D. "Social Support and Mortality in an Elderly Community Population." *American Journal of Epidemiology*, 1982, *115*(5), 684–694.

Buckingham, M., and Coffman, C. *First Break All the Rules: What the World's Greatest Managers Do Differently*. New York: Simon & Schuster, 1999.

Gerteis, M., Edgman-Levitan, S., Daley, J., and Delbanco, T. (eds.). *Through the Patient's Eyes: Understanding and Promoting Patient-Centered Care*. San Francisco: Jossey-Bass, 1993.

Kamarack, T., Manuck, S., and Jennings, J. "Social Support Reduces Cardiovascular Reactivity to Psychological Challenge: A Laboratory Model." *Psychosomatic Medicine*, 1990, *52*, 42–58.

Kovach, K. A. "What Motivates Employees? Workers and Supervisors Give Different Answers." *Business Horizons*, Sep./Oct., 1987, *30*(5), 58.

Lepore, S., Mata Allen, K., and Evans, G. "Social Support Lowers Cardiovascular Reactivity in an Acute Stressor." *Psychosomatic Medicine*, 1993, *55*, 518–524.

Levering, R. Keynote address, Building a Positive Work Environment conference, Coronado, Calif., Nov. 15, 2001.

Lindheim, R. "Criteria for Creating Environments That Promote Caring." Proceedings from the Symposium: "Environments for Humanized Health Care," Berkeley, Calif., Mar. 1979.

Lindheim, R., "Birthing Centers and Hospices: Reclaiming Birth and Death." *Annual Review of Public Health,* 1981, *2,* 1–29.

Lindheim, R. "New Design Parameters for Healthy Places." *Places,* 1985, *2*(4), 17–27.

Lindheim, R., and Syme, L. "Environments, People, and Health." *Annual Review of Public Health,* 1983, *4,* 335–359.

Martin, D., and others. "Randomized Trial of a Patient-Centered Hospital Unit." *Patient Education and Counseling,* 1998 (34), pp. 125–133.

Ornish, D. *Love and Survival.* New York: Harper Perennial, 1998.

Press Ganey Associates. "One Million Patients Have Spoken: Who Will Listen?" *The Satisfaction Monitor,* 1999.

Reynolds, P., and Kaplan, G. "Social Connections and Risk for Cancer: Prospective Evidence from the Alameda County Study." *Behavioral Medicine,* 1990, *16*(3), 101–110.

Spiegel, D. *Living Beyond Limits.* New York: Fawcett, 1993.

Wiklund, I., and others. "Prognostic Importance of Somatic and Psychosocial Variables After a First Myocardial Infarction." *American Journal of Epidemiology,* 1988, *128*(4), 786–795.

Williams, R., and others. "Prognostic Importance of Social and Economic Resources Among Medically Treated Patients with Angiographically Documented Coronary Artery Disease." *Journal of the American Medical Association,* 1992, *267*(4), 520–524.

2

Informing and Empowering Diverse Populations

Consumer Health Libraries and Patient Education

Candace Ford and Laura Gilpin

In recent years, health care has begun to refocus on caring for the whole person—body, mind, and spirit. The *mind* often refers to emotional or psychosocial health—both essential aspects of well-being. But other aspects of the mind are the mental and intellectual needs, which are vital to recovering from an acute illness or managing a chronic condition and promoting and maintaining health. Especially with the complexity of today's health care options, information and education are essential if patients and consumers are to become active partners in their care.

The Vital Role for Health Information Services

Access to health and medical information has always been one of the cornerstones of the Planetree model. Planetree was founded in 1978, at a time when information was scarce for patients and consumers. Most medical libraries were closed to the public, the Internet was not available, and medical information about the patient was routinely withheld. Nurses were instructed not to tell patients their vital signs, and hospitals made it difficult for patients to review their own medical records. As passive recipients of health care, patients and consumers were perceived to have no need for information. Yet one of the major complaints of health care consumers throughout the years has been lack of information (Gerteis, Edgman-Levitan, Daley, and Delbanco, 1993).

Although times have changed dramatically, the need for accurate, unbiased, and balanced information is no less important. Rather than a dearth of information, consumers now face a deluge. The sheer volume of health information now available to the public can be overwhelming, leaving people confused by conflicting messages. Direct-to-consumer advertising of prescription drugs and heavily marketed books and authors can blur the public's perception of reliability. Highly promoted commercial Web sites may be better known than government, academic, and professional sources. Hype and popularity may be perceived by the public as accuracy and efficacy.

While information is proliferating, professional guidance is in short supply. Because of changes in reimbursement, many physicians have less time to spend answering patients' questions and explaining diagnoses and treatment options. Short lengths of stay for hospitalized patients and increased staffing demands give nurses little time for teaching.

Increasingly, some people are realizing that they need to do their own research to explore all available treatment options, not just standard protocols or those that may be covered by their insurance plan. Despite the technical difficulty of medical texts for most readers, motivated consumers can be remarkably dedicated in their efforts to comprehend the professional literature for their particular concern. As one consumer health librarian observed, "Anyone can learn to understand a few nine-syllable medical terms when it's their son's illness, or their mother's, or their own."

However strong their personal motivation to learn about health, for people whose English or literacy skills are weak, even an article or pamphlet, much less navigating the World Wide Web, may be intimidating. A significant number of people in the United States have limited reading and writing skills. Some immigrants have limited English abilities or prefer to learn about medical issues in their primary language. And among American-born English-speaking adults, at least 25 percent cannot read or write sufficiently to sign medical consent forms or read medication labels. According to the National Academy on an Aging Society (1999), health literacy issues cost the American health care system approximately $73 billion annually.

For underserved populations, lack of access to relevant health information in any format remains an immense barrier. For much of the general population who have access to computers and on-line services, locating and evaluating health information on the Internet can be problematic. In 2002, as various studies compared and contrasted the comprehensiveness and accuracy of popular medical Web sites, over seventy million people reported going on-line for health information (Fox and Rainie, 2002).

But many people—not only those with poor English or literacy skills—have difficulty using the new information technologies. This is particularly true for older adults, who often have multiple health issues. Whereas some are extremely savvy users of the Internet, many seniors have difficulty manipulating a mouse or keyboard, much less performing an on-line search. Even among people who are comfortable using computers, many lack the experience and in-depth training to find and evaluate Internet health sources. No matter how many computers are purchased for home use or donated to community centers, many people need training, guidance, and practice to skillfully obtain the health information they need from a computer.

With more members of the public searching for current and reliable medical information, and with many of these people ill-prepared to take on such a search, it is clear that consumer health information services and patient education programs are more vital than ever. Planetree's core values of patient-centered care and community responsiveness provide an ideal framework for helping people find accurate, balanced, and unbiased information.

Consumer Health Libraries

When faced with an acute illness, Planetree founder Angelica Thieriot could not find the information she needed to understand the medical condition that resulted in her hospitalization. At that time, hospital libraries were closed to patients and families, public libraries offered few current health resources, and most academic medical center libraries were reluctant to make their collections and services available to community members.

In response to her frustrations, Thieriot envisioned taking the best from public and medical libraries to create an innovative hybrid. To this new type of community library, Thieriot added two vital elements: personalized assistance and an environment that was conducive to both learning and healing. With support from health care and community leaders, the concept for a consumer medical library began to build, with fundraising and grant dollars helping to underwrite the first Planetree library.

The Planetree Health Resource Center opened in San Francisco in July 1981, in a space carefully designed to be unintimidating. Its rectangular open space had high ceilings, colorful works of art, and fresh-cut flowers. Natural lighting provided by large windows overlooked colorful flower boxes and landscaping. The comfortable furniture included wooden tables and a variety of chairs to choose from. There was also a counter with stools so that people who were uncomfortable sitting (for example, from back injuries or pregnancy) could stand while researching. There were the typical public library amenities, and Planetree featured a children's toy and book corner. The photocopier relied on the honor system; no one was turned away if he or she lacked the ten cents a page to pay for copies. A health bookstore allowed people to purchase popular and, at that time, hard-to-find books, audiotapes, videotapes, and self-help products—for example, relaxation tapes, a baby food grinder, an ear scope, or a gum massager.

The collection was remarkable in its breadth and depth of health and medical information. It included lay-oriented books next to current medical texts, as well as alternative therapy information and conventional medicine classics. A key element in this new community agency was the assistance offered to each patron by the staff and volunteers, whose compassionate approach helped to both empower and comfort people as they faced the medical concerns of themselves and their families.

San Francisco and surrounding communities embraced this maverick concept—that consumers could become well informed about their individual health issues through a new type of library that was free and open to the public. Many studies have shown that better-informed patients often have better outcomes, but such conclusions were based on specific common conditions and standardized educational materials. Providing patients and community members with a true research center for their own in-depth study was a new direction, which began some fifteen years before the explosion of information on the Internet. The medical field took note of this very different medical library and its pioneering principles that recognized the importance of individuals taking responsibility for their own health and health care. As the first Planetree library served walk-in patrons, plus hundreds from around the country through a then-unique research-by-mail service, Thieriot continued her work of bringing changes to the medical world.

Hallmarks of Planetree Libraries and Resource Centers

The Planetree health resource center concept has been emulated by health care organizations around the country. While most are established as special services within hospital settings, others are stand-alone centers within communities or even in shopping malls, where heavy "consumer traffic" guarantees exposure to, and utilization by, a wide variety of individuals.

In a Planetree library setting, an inexperienced patron may need considerable assistance and suggestions from the staff on where to start his or her research, whereas a library-savvy patron may find the comprehensive collection so well organized that self-directed searching is a pleasure. Each Planetree resource center is developed to reflect the diverse information needs of its community, including education levels, languages other than English, and learning styles. Planetree collections reflect their local community's cultural approaches to healing by including information on therapeutic modalities such as traditional Chinese medicine and Native American healing. The Planetree core concept of choice—for patients and their families and for community members—is demonstrated by each library's community assessment and by the provision of a wide range of resources.

Responding to the needs of all community members, Planetree libraries in areas with large immigrant populations include bilingual or multilingual health materials. A Planetree resource center includes information on medical diagnoses and treatment options, both conventional and complementary. Caregiving, coping with chronic illness, and life processes from fertility issues to death and dying are part of the collection. The importance of mental health, stress management, and relationships, as well as informed choices in diet, nutrition, and exercise, are also part of the collection. These myriad consumer health issues are addressed through lay books, medical texts, technical journals, newsletters, materials for adult new readers, and audiovisual media and computer services.

One element common to Planetree libraries is their unique organization of all these materials. The Planetree classification scheme was created for the original library when it became clear that the medical information world had no scheme that would help a lay person know that *heart attack* and *myocardial infarction* refer to the same life-threatening event. The Planetree scheme, which has had several revisions, has been used by hundreds of agencies and other libraries that want a consumer-oriented way to organize their print, audiovisual, and on-line materials. A health collection arranged by the Planetree classification scheme makes intuitive sense to a lay person because it is a logical ordering of like topics, from broad to specific categories. It is very browsable and increases the likelihood of finding a related helpful book. Sometimes a person makes profound discoveries from browsing the unit or resource center collection. This is especially true for lifestyle and self-care information, such as stress triggers and coping strategies. Ease of use for community members is important, since some people are shy about making known their concerns to others and only want to do self-directed research. The classification scheme is an important tool that facilitates a patron's work and supports the empowerment process.

However, among collections of health information resources, it is not the collection itself but the connections between people that sets Planetree apart. Planetree library reference services are provided by expert and dedicated paid and volunteer staff members. Librarians, library assistants, health educators, community members, and students provide individuals with unbiased help in locating the information they seek. With years of experience in the "reference interview" and listening with what social workers call "the third ear," consumer health librarians become specialists in serving the vastly different information needs of the general community. Medical librarians accustomed to working with health care professionals remark on how different it is to help worried, fearful clientele. "The patron's visit is often lengthy and often requires more than one interaction with library staff. . . . It is this poignant contact with patrons that makes consumer health library staff so passionate about their work"(Flake, forthcoming).

Planetree library services rely on the talents, commitment, and efforts of volunteers in all areas of the operation—from advisory board members to gardeners. Volunteers are often the first line of reference assistance that a patron may encounter for library orientation and direction. Volunteers receive in-depth reference service training by library professionals that emphasizes the importance of teaching patrons how to access medical information. Volunteers learn that they cannot provide advice, interpretation, or opinions; nor can they share their personal medical histories. They are taught to access the library professional to provide backup assistance regarding reference services and library policies.

Planetree institutions are known for encouraging the public to be well informed and empowered health care consumers, but it is the staff members of the Planetree libraries that enable patients to make informed decisions about their personal health care and well-being. Each patient adopts a unique set of decision-making criteria to which the library staff must be sensitive. Library staff members respect an individual's wish *not* to be an active participant in his or her medical decision making as much as they respect that individual's right to be in total control of his or her health care decisions.

In recent years, computerized information sources have become an integral part of all libraries, and various computer services are now expected by the public. Planetree resource centers have initiated the service of training patrons to effectively search the Internet for health and medical information, as detailed in an article coauthored by the librarian and Planetree manager at Highline Community Hospital in Burien, Washington. Maksirisombat and Taylor (2002) also note that cooperative purchasing of Web-based products "can help libraries obtain more resources than they would be able to afford on their own limited budgets" (p. 59). Additional full-text articles for patrons are provided through Planetree libraries' participation in on-line interlibrary loan services.

Sometimes the most helpful information does not come from a book or a Web site but from another person who has the same health concern or diagnosis. Planetree libraries facilitate access to such information by helping people find contacts for local and national health organizations and support groups. In addition to contact information in telephone books, directories, journals, and other publications, the DIRLINE section of the National Library of Medicine (http://dirline.nlm.nih.gov/) updates information on many such associations. Some Planetree libraries maintain a "consumer health network," which enables an individual to share information and support with another patron who is available by phone, by e-mail, or in person. Article files, a component of some Planetree libraries, offer selections from incoming medical journals, magazines, and newsletters. Articles of particular educational value are copied and organized by specific diagnosis or health topic. For example, the file on scleroderma is found in the drawer of connective tissue diseases, and articles on seasonal affective disorders are located behind the major heading of "mental health and illness." Having a selection of articles from many different sources is immediately gratifying to someone who is starting to research a medical condition.

Some resource centers sell health-related books and gifts and offer health lectures and classes. St. Joseph Regional Medical Center in Mishawaka, Indiana sponsors "To Your Health," which features a health retail store and classrooms, as well as a reference library. In addition to traditional health education offerings, clients can sign up for unusual classes, such as "Natural Lawn Care" or "Eccentricity: Fostering Health Through Individuality and Creativity." At the health shop, merchandise includes yoga mats, stress relief videos, walking kits, exercise balls, and natural cosmetics and aromatherapies.

Variety of Planetree Libraries

Although the hallmarks of Planetree libraries represent a cohesive, well-grounded philosophy, the clientele, settings, and locations vary widely. Some Planetree-affiliated libraries focus on serving the general public, often with special services for hospital patients and their families. Others are medical libraries that serve physicians and other health care professionals, as well as patients and community members. Some Planetree resource centers are housed in charming Victorians or other noninstitutional settings. Other libraries are located within the hospital that funds them, as part of a main welcoming lobby, near family waiting rooms, or in a renovated hospital wing. Others are across town from their institutional sponsors, including one in forty-two hundred square feet of the largest shopping center in the region.

There are two types of library affiliations within the Planetree national network. The majority of Planetree libraries are operated by Planetree hospitals. Several years ago, Planetree created a library-only affiliation at the request of hospitals and community health agencies that wanted to affiliate with an established consumer health information network without full Planetree hospital affiliation status. The Mercy Health Resource Library at St. John's Regional Medical Center in Joplin, Missouri, one of the first library-only Planetree affiliates, eventually helped facilitate its hospital's interest in becoming part of the Planetree alliance as well, with the inpatient psychiatric unit serving as the initial Planetree hospital unit. In California's Napa Valley, a library affiliate operates as part of Queen of the Valley Hospital's department of community outreach, supporting such efforts as HIV treatment and education, cancer case management, and prenatal care. The health library also provides assistance to a community center serving Latino families, which includes setting up a bilingual library for children and adults, which features a health section.

Outreach: Taking Health Information Services Outside the Library

Led by library-only and hospital affiliates alike, health education efforts out in the community are in place throughout the Planetree network. The Cancer Education Center of the Greenville Hospital System, a Planetree affiliate in Greenville, South Carolina, takes a multitude of cancer resources to health fairs at large corporations, assisted living facilities, and community centers. Back at the hospital, the center holds community prostate screenings, including PSA blood tests and a urologist's exam. The cancer center's library supports patients and families by delivering packets of requested material to patients' rooms.

In Derby, Connecticut, Griffin Hospital's "Mobile Health Resource Center" makes frequent trips out into the community to offer blood pressure screenings and a minicollection of health books and tapes to lend and pamphlets to give away. Staffed by parish nurses and volunteers, the van also has an Internet-connected computer available for teaching people about effective health searching on-line. Often this interaction is the first time a community member hears about the much larger consumer health library available to all at Griffin Hospital.

Several Planetree libraries tailor powerful outreach services for specific groups, realizing that for some members of the community, the concept of a public library, much less one focused on health, is unfamiliar. By partnering with other agencies and developing branch libraries and satellite collections, the Planetree library in San Jose has developed effective models for taking health information services to where people "live, shop, learn, and pray." These branch libraries are funded through special grants for reaching underserved communities and are staffed with part-time bilingual library assistants. Oversight of the collection, training for the staff and volunteers, and the submission of new grants are among the responsibilities of the main Planetree affiliate. Working with patrons in these branches has demonstrated firsthand that attempting to use the Internet is frustrating for recent immigrants who are new to computers, American culture, and the English language. In response, the Planetree San Jose library Web site (http://www.planetreesanjose.org) includes an extensive section: "En español." Designed for monolingual Spanish speakers, it features an extensive list of evaluated links in Spanish, offered in an easy-to-use format. For English-only librarians and health professionals who serve Spanish-speaking patients and families, there is a mirror home page of that section in English.

People who live in rural areas also benefit from special outreach efforts. The primary service area of the Mid-Columbia Medical Center in The Dalles, Oregon, has nearly fifty-seven hundred square miles, which requires patrons to drive as much as an hour to reach the medical and resource centers. In addition to giving talks at local groups throughout the area, the resource center staff's presentation to school district officials led to a required in-service for area teachers—at the Planetree Health Resource Center. Outreach to classes has continued, as has participation in the annual

Teacher Fair. Branch libraries at an area clinic and an oncology center, as well as new technologies, also help meet "the difficulties of distance and geography" in providing health information services (Spatz, 2000).

Promoting Health Information Services to the Community

Wherever the Planetree information services are located, publicizing what they have to offer requires ongoing effort and creative strategies. By the time a person is in the hospital, the urge to research may have diminished because the illness and healing processes themselves require the patient's full attention. It is often more effective to market information services to family members and visiting friends than to the patient, especially with a shortened length of stay and the higher acuity so common among patients today.

In the general community, people may be glad to hear about the availability of a health library but do not need it at that time. McCall (1999) suggests that "people do not typically pay attention to CHI [consumer health information] services until they need health information." Therefore, libraries need ongoing, effective promotion of their services "so that when people do need health information they will see immediately where to get it" (p. 4). McCall has compiled a multitude of techniques for promoting libraries to both consumers and health professionals.

One effective yet no-cost technique was employed by a library affiliate, which prevailed upon the city to erect "Health Library" signs in both directions on a nearby busy road. Those signs and a prominent book drop at the curb also help attract passers-by, who come in saying, "I didn't know about your library and my mother was just diagnosed." Getting out the message about services is an ongoing and multifaceted effort. Other useful techniques are outlined on the NN/LM Consumer Health Library outreach sections of their Web site (http://nnlm.gov/scr/conhlth/manualidx.htm). The Consumer and Patient Health Information Section (CAPHIS) of the National Library of Medicine also has a robust Web site (http://www.caphis.mlanet.org), which is useful to both novice and experienced librarians.

Promotional activities may not relate to the patron directly but, rather, to primary referral groups. Public libraries and health care professionals often suggest that a visit to a health library would be helpful. The Harris Methodist library affiliate of Texas Health Resources formalized its relationships with the Dallas–Ft. Worth public library system. When a participating public library is unable to fill a patron's health information needs, the librarian contacts the Planetree affiliate. Health library staff members later interview the patron over the phone to create a tailored information packet, which is mailed to him or her. The directors of the public library system have committed to training their staff about this valuable service from the medical library and are promoting their Planetree library affiliation with the targeted distribution of brochures.

Although referrals by other library and health care colleagues are effective, surveys of Planetree libraries consistently show that the most common referral source is by word of mouth from very satisfied patrons.

Funding and the Purpose of Consumer Health Libraries

The greatest funding challenge for a community health library is to cover ongoing operating and administrative expenses. Grants are available to reach underserved patients and community members; hospitals and health systems are eager to fund a new service that will help to distinguish them from their competitors in the eyes of potential patients and medical staff members. But enlightened self-interest and "side door marketing" can wear thin when the economic realities of operating a hospital in today's hostile environment force budgets to be scrutinized. For consumer health libraries, the challenge in funding is not to start but to continue.

The most successfully funded consumer health libraries may have several revenue streams, but it is essential that their primary funding be an independent line item on the budget of their institutional sponsors. Donations from "grateful patrons" and direct mail campaigns are often highly successful, as are special events and other community collaborations, but they are insufficient to fund ongoing operations. Hospitals and health agencies support nonrevenue-producing departments, such as consumer health libraries, for many reasons. The desire to enhance the health of the individuals and families of the community in which they operate is part of the mission statement of most hospitals and health systems. Therefore, operating a consumer health library is viewed as being consistent with the hospital's core mission. Sponsoring institutions realize that neither philanthropic support nor the use of statistics can measure the worth of a Planetree library's complex and personal service. In the hands of consumers, health information ensures avenues to better health, and it even saves lives.

Planetree Patient and Family Education

Frequently, when people become patients, their educational needs change. Some patients may have taken their health for granted until an unexpected health crisis refocused their attention. And some patients are well educated and informed, arriving with computer searches in hand, ready to discuss the latest treatment options with their physicians. Family members, who are vital to providing care for patients at home, may feel unprepared to take on the role of caregiver. Given the diverse educational needs of patients and their families, health care professionals at hospitals, clinics, community health centers, and physicians' offices are challenged to meet those needs (Giloth, 1993). The Institute of Medicine (Committee on Quality of Health Care in America, 2001) lists "access to information" as a primary principle in creating health care for the twenty-first century.

Since the opening of the first Planetree model unit in 1985, Planetree's goal for hospitals has been to go beyond simply providing quality medical care to creating an environment in which patients and their families are offered the tools, skills, and knowledge they need to be active partners in their care. Illness is seen as an educational opportunity. Patients, who may have few resources at home, are brought together with numerous health professionals, including nurses, physicians, pharmacists, dietitians, physical therapists, social workers, and chaplains, who are willing to share their knowledge in an environment conducive to learning. The Planetree model for education is both patient-centered and patient-driven, encouraging patients to ask questions and participate in the decision-making process, enabling them to direct their own care. Many Planetree hospitals have expanded the traditional protocols of providing standardized educational resources to offering information based on patients' interests and requests. Many patients, for instance, have questions about lifestyle changes, coping skills, or the illnesses of other family members. Highline Community Hospital no longer uses the traditional term *patient education*, instead referring to its program as patient and family information.

Despite the widespread availability of information on the Internet and in the community, and despite recommendations by the Joint Commission on Accreditation of Healthcare Organizations to provide patients with health and medical information, patient focus groups and surveys reveal that many hospital education programs are failing to meet patients' needs and expectations (Gerteis, Edgman-Levitan, Daley, and Delbanco, 1993). Although many facilities have goals of providing education, the realities of today's health care environment present numerous challenges and barriers. With the diversity of patients' educational needs and high acuity, as well as tight budgets and low staffing, education is rarely a daily priority. Too often, patient teaching is left until the day of discharge, when the patient and her family may be distracted and unable to concentrate on the information being given.

There are also lingering attitudes among some health professionals that patients do not want information. Others believe that if patients are well informed, they might refuse medications, treatments, or diagnostic tests, or they would be more likely to question their practitioners' judgment. There is also the fear that educated patients are more likely to take legal action against the physician or hospital. However, studies support the experience at Planetree hospitals, which is that knowledgeable patients are not more likely to ignore their physicians' advice; nor are they more likely to file lawsuits. On the contrary, it is a lack of information that prompts some angry patients to sue (Lichtstein, Materson, and Spicer, 1999; Colon, 2002).

There are also concerns that patient and family education is expensive. Some aspects of a comprehensive education program can increase costs, such as additional nurses' wages if they spend more time teaching, or an added salary if a patient and family educator is hired. However, many effective aspects of an education program add very little to a hospital budget. Although difficult to document, education programs may offer significant cost savings by decreasing the length of stay and preventing complications and readmissions (Webber, 1990). Increased patient satisfaction in a competitive market and the potential for decreased litigation may help offset costs for educational services.

Elements of a Patient and Family Education Program

Although Planetree hospitals vary in their implementation of the Planetree model, many have incorporated the following elements into their patient and family education programs.

Educational Relationships

One of the most important aspects of an educational environment is the relationship among the patient, the family, and those who provide the care. Two-way communication is essential with nurses and other staff members who are educating and informing as well as asking and listening. Staff members play a vital role in creating an atmosphere conducive to learning throughout the patient's stay. Patients and families often need encouragement from the staff to ask questions and seek information. Unless encouraged, some patients are reluctant to ask questions, for fear of offending physicians or staff members.

Planetree hospitals differ widely in identifying who will be accountable for providing education and responding to the patient's and family's informational needs. Many see staff nurses as the primary educators because of their accessibility to patients. Other hospitals, such as Mid-Columbia Medical Center and Highline Community Hospital, employ information and education coordinators, often expanding the role to include coordination of the care partner program. At Mid-Columbia, the Planetree coordinator visits all patients at least once to inquire about educational needs. At Highline, the Planetree coordinator rarely sees patients but instead works with the staff to identify resources for each specialty area and to find ways to integrate patient and family education into daily care.

Sometimes, the best teachers are other patients and families who can share similar experiences about coping with illness. Creating opportunities for interaction between patients and between families provides educational opportunities that few health care professionals can offer. By having a kitchen on the unit that draws people together, or an arts program that offers concerts and other events, Planetree hospitals enable patients and families to support one another and exchange information about coping and caregiving.

The Open-Chart Policy

One of the most valuable, least expensive educational resources is the patient's own medical record. Encouraging a patient to read his or her own chart helps create an environment of trust and openness, often initiating a dialogue between patients and caregivers (Grange, Renvoize, and Pinder, 1998).

At most Planetree hospitals, a growing number of patients choose to read their medical record when informed by the staff of this option. A recent survey by Planetree of eight affiliates with open-chart policies found that on average approximately 30 percent of patients are actively encouraged to read their chart. Of these, over 40 percent choose to. The first several times patients read their record, nurses review the information with them to answer questions and explain abbreviations. A frequently heard comment from patients after reading the chart is, "My doctor has already told me this." The medical record provides reassurance that information is not being withheld.

Most patients who read their medical record read it only once. A few read it daily, reviewing orders and test results. One patient with severe liver damage was able to track improvements in his liver function tests while he was hospitalized and not consuming alcohol. Seeing the evidence that his liver was recovering offered him hope that changing his lifestyle could improve his prognosis. This was the impetus for his requesting information about joining Alcoholics Anonymous.

In addition to reading their chart, some patients choose to write about their perspective in the Patients' Progress Notes, which, at their request, becomes a permanent part of the medical record. To protect confidentiality, only the patient has access to his or her own medical record. If the patient would like a family member to have access to the chart, he or she can sign a form, releasing medical information to the designated person.

An open medical record is also a valuable asset in risk management. Patients have prevented numerous errors by noticing that important information, such as allergies, was missing from the record or by pointing out discrepancies in medication orders.

The Self-Medication Program

A self-medication program provides an opportunity for patients to begin taking responsibility for their own care while they are in the hospital and have the support of nurses, physicians, and pharmacists. Any patient who is mentally alert and interested in learning about his or her medications is encouraged, but not required, to participate in the program. For patients who have been taking medications successfully at home, a self-medication program reinforces

their ability to manage their own care. For patients new to a regimen, learning about medications in a monitored environment gives
them the knowledge and confidence that they will manage successfully at home. Because of high acuity and short lengths of stay,
many patients may be unable to participate, although rehabilitation
units and other areas where patients stay longer and are more alert
are ideal settings for this program.

The Care Coordination Conference

To encourage good communication, at many Planetree hospitals,
a nurse schedules a care coordination conference, usually within
twenty-four hours of a patient's admission. This brief meeting,
often lasting no longer than ten minutes, includes the physician,
the nurse, the patient, and, ideally, a member or members of the
patient's family. The purpose of the conference is to clarify the goals
and expectations of the treatment plan. The expected day of discharge and discharge planning may also be discussed so that educational needs can be anticipated and resources can be provided.
The care coordination conference is a useful way to ensure that
all members of the health care team, including the patient and
family, are involved in the decisions determining the patient's care
and have congruent expectations.

Many physicians are initially concerned about the difficulty of
scheduling these conferences or the time that may be involved.
Once the routine is established, many find that the conferences save
time, as they facilitate communicating directly with all involved. If
it is impossible to bring the group together for a conference, the
information is exchanged informally, although the active participation of the patient, whenever possible, is essential.

The Physical Environment

The environment can play a key role in creating an atmosphere
conducive to learning. Traditional hospital design grew out of an
old paradigm in which information was not readily available to

patients or their families. Nurses sat behind high counters, often with glass partitions, making it difficult for patients to ask questions or request information.

A well-designed hospital not only creates a comfortable, home-like environment; it also provides spaces that promote and enhance learning. Kitchens, lounges, and activity rooms create opportunities for information sharing and educational interactions. At Mid-Columbia Medical Center, traditional nurses' stations have been transformed into open *communication centers*, where patients and families can ask questions and access information.

Satellite Libraries

Another type of space that facilitates learning at many Planetree hospitals is the unit or satellite library. These smaller libraries, in easily accessible areas, provide a range of educational resources, often focusing on the specific needs of the unit, such as information on cancer or cardiology. Depending on space, they often include books and pamphlets, audiotapes and videotapes, and a computer for on-line searching. A copier and printer enable patients and families to take information home with them.

Information Packets

For hospitals with Planetree health resource centers, personalized information packets are offered to patients on any health or medical topic. Upon a patient's admission or at the request of a nurse, library staff members and volunteers create a packet of information to be delivered to the patient's room or mailed to the patient's home. A packet may also include information on local support groups and complementary modalities relevant to the patient's condition and/or interests.

The personalized information packet service provides a valuable resource for nurses, particularly when they are asked questions that they are initially unprepared to answer. For example, when a surgical patient asks about her granddaughter's heart defect, the nurse can request an information packet to review later with the patient.

Educational Materials

Fact sheets, available from a variety of sources, offer information on common diagnoses, tests and procedures, and medications. Ideally, fact sheets are written in patient-empowering language, avoiding commands ("Do this. . . . Don't do that. . . .") and providing explanations and rationale. At many hospitals, fact sheets are available in various locations and through the hospital's information system so that the appropriate titles can be printed on demand from any nurses' station. Some hospitals also offer copies of fact sheets in wall racks to anyone who is interested in them, supporting the message that access to information and education is valued and promoted.

The Planetree Book Cart

A Planetree book cart for patient and family education is not the typical hospital book cart containing fiction and magazines; instead, it is a rolling collection of print and audio materials that focus on healing, relaxation, humor, recovery, and inspiration. Often staffed by volunteers, a Planetree book cart may also include books and illustrated booklets on specific conditions. Items borrowed by patients or their families are easily returned to the nurse's station in specially marked envelopes so that library staff members or volunteers can return them to the book cart. "Takeaways" may also be offered from the cart, such as a list of a medical librarian's favorite health and medical Web sites—for more effective on-line searches.

Book cart services can be particularly effective for hospitals with multiple campuses. The Planetree Health Library in San Jose provides a book cart service to its sponsor, Good Samaritan Hospital, located across town. The Planetree book cart provides information and inspiration to patients and families at the main campus, introducing them to the in-depth services of the Planetree health library, located on a specialty campus.

Summary

Despite the spectacular achievements of modern medicine in diagnosing, treating, and curing illness, technological advances alone cannot create health. Preventing illness and promoting health can only be achieved through the active participation of each health care consumer. And participation is predicated on information and knowledge.

If the goal of health care is *health* and well-being, access to information and education must be valued and supported. Few question a hospital's decision to purchase the most advanced imaging machine or the latest piece of surgical equipment. Yet consumer health libraries and patient and family education programs are rarely seen as priorities. Perhaps the greatest achievement of modern medicine will be not only to successfully diagnose and treat illness but also to embrace informed consumers in the care delivery process and in the promotion of health and well-being.

References

Colon, V. F. "Ten Ways to Reduce Medical Malpractice Exposure." *The Physician Executive*, 2002, *28*(2), 16–18.

Committee on Quality of Health Care in America, Institute of Medicine. *Crossing the Quality Chasm: A New Health System for the Twenty-First Century*. Washington, D.C.: National Academy Press, 2001.

Flake, D. "A Dozen Excellent Consumer Health Libraries." In A. Rees (ed.), *The Consumer Health Information Source Book* (7th ed.). Westport, Conn.: Greenwood Press, forthcoming.

Fox, S., and Rainie, L. "Vital Decisions: How Internet Users Decide What Information to Trust When They or Their Loved Ones Are Sick." [http://www.pewinternet.org/reports/toc.asp?Report=59]. May 22, 2002.

Gerteis, M., Edgman-Levitan, S., Daley, J., and Delbanco, T. (eds.). *Through the Patient's Eyes: Understanding and Promoting Patient-Centered Care*. San Francisco, Jossey-Bass, 1993.

Giloth, B. (ed.). *Managing Hospital-Based Patient Education*. Chicago: American Hospital Association Publishing, 1993.

Grange, A., Renvoize, E., and Pinder, J. "Patients' Rights to Access Their Healthcare Records." *Nursing Standard*, 1998, *13*(6), 41–42.

Lichtstein, D., Materson, B., and Spicer, D. "Reducing the Risk of Malpractice Claims." *Hospital Practice*, 1999, 34(7), 69–72, 75–76, 79.

Maksirisombat, I., and Taylor, D. "Internet Access in a Consumer Health Library." *Journal of Hospital Librarianship*, 2002, 2(1), 57–62.

McCall, K. (compiler). *Introduction to Marketing the Consumer Health Information Service: MLA DocKit #12*. Chicago, Ill.: Medical Library Association, 1999.

National Academy on an Aging Society. "Low Health Literacy Skills Contribute to Higher Utilization of Health Care Services." [http://www.agingsociety.org/healthlit.htm]. 1999.

Spatz, M. A.. "Providing Consumer Health Information in the Rural Setting: Planetree Health Resource Center's Approach." *Bulletin of the Medical Library Association*, 2000, 88(4), 382–388. [http://www.pubmedcentral.gov/articlerender.fcgi?tool=pubmed&pubmedid=11055307].

Webber, G. "Patient Education: A Review of the Issues." *Medical Care*, 1990, 28(11), 1089–1103.

3

Healing Partnerships

The Importance of Including Family and Friends

Susan Edgman-Levitan

The Institute of Medicine report *Crossing the Quality Chasm* (Committee on Quality of Health Care in America, 2001) is a call for the complete transformation of the existing health care system. This report urges the building of bridges from where we are currently to a new system of care that is, at its very core, patient- and family-centered. Specifically, the report maps the design of a health care system that is safe, effective, patient-centered, timely, efficient, and equitable. The definition of patient-centered care in *Crossing the Quality Chasm* was adapted from the work of the Picker Institute in Boston (Gerteis, Edgman-Levitan, Daley, and Delbanco, 1993). Based on information from patient and family focus groups and data from thousands of patient surveys conducted by the Picker Institute, the dimensions of care that patients and families most value are

- Respect for patient preferences and involvement in decision making

- Access to care

- Coordination of care

- Information and education

- Physical comfort

- Emotional support

- Involvement of family and friends

- Continuity—transition from the hospital or other settings of care to home

Involving and caring for the patient's family and friends is a critical dimension. In the Planetree model, the family is much more than "next of kin." *Family* means whoever the patient recognizes as significant.

Anyone who has ever been sick, even if only for a few days, understands the importance of family members and friends in the healing process. Favorite foods prepared "just the way you like it," a cold compress to the forehead, and the reassuring presence of a loved one sitting quietly at your side have an immeasurable power to comfort the body and fortify the spirit. In her chapter in *Through the Patient's Eyes* (Gerteis, Edgman-Levitan, Daley, and Delbanco, 1993), Beth Ellers presents a compelling argument for the importance of caring for the patient and family as a family.

Family members, close friends, and "significant others" can have a far greater impact on patients' experience of illness, and on their long-term health and happiness, than any health care professional. Friends and relatives take care of patients, especially when they are home. They offer love and encouragement. They may cook meals, look after children, handle the shopping, pay bills, or take on any of the myriad responsibilities of daily life that a sick person cannot fulfill. They often convince the person to seek medical help and then steer them through the receptionists, triage nurses, doctors, billing and insurance offices, and other hurdles of the healthcare system. They are the eyes and ears that watch over patients and report what they see to doctors and nurses. They remind patients to take medications

and follow treatment regimens. And through their own
behavior they profoundly influence the lifetime habits
that affect the patient's well-being over the long run.

The Picker Institute conducted focus groups with doctors and
nurses about their perspective on the dimensions of patient-centered
care. It was clear from these groups that doctors and other clinical
staff members find families frustrating, annoying, and difficult. Few
seemed to comprehend how their negative perceptions affect patients
and their families. The dissonance between the perspective of families and that of the hospital staff can be enormous. Research suggests
that patients prefer having family involvement in care more often
than what traditionally occurs in practice (Botelho, Lue, and Fiscella,
1996). In an exercise often conducted at Planetree staff retreats, participants are encouraged to put themselves in the place of a hospitalized patient. Overwhelmingly, they identify access to family and
friends as the most important element of that imagined experience.

Many patients in the hospital are anxious, uncomfortable, disori-
ented, and afraid. They want trusted family members to listen to
information and help them make important decisions. The 1989
Picker national study of the health care experience of recently discharged patients and their families found that family members value
emotional support, involvement in discharge planning, and involvement in decision making. The study also revealed considerable dissatisfaction with discharge planning and family participation in the
patients' care (vom Eigen and others, 1999). Low income, emergency
admissions, and poor patient health status were associated with higher
problem scores for family members. When the patient's regular doctor delivered care, the families reported higher levels of satisfaction. It
is a simple fact that families need and want the same things that
patients do: information, emotional support, and respect (vom Eigen
and others, 1999). Yet many staff members and physicians feel that
families are dysfunctional when family members question staff
actions or persist in trying to meet patient needs.

When hospital staff members are asked to list the attributes of the "perfect patient and family," their response is usually a passive patient with no family. The ideal patient is described as one who does not ask questions, never rings the call bell, does exactly what he or she is told, and has no visible family members or friends to advocate on his or her behalf. Which is more "dysfunctional"—the family trying to support their loved one or the staff member who pretends they don't exist and aren't important?

If we think about what patients and families experience in most health care settings, we find that being a patient is the closest most people get to the experience of being in prison. Patients are stripped of control, their clothes are taken away, they have little say over their schedule—when they eat, bathe, or even go to the bathroom—and they are deliberately separated from their family and friends. Health care professionals control all of the information about their patients' bodies and access to the people who can answer questions and connect them with helpful resources. From the family's perspective, they are treated more as intruders than as loved ones. At best, they are "visitors." But who are the real visitors in the patient's life—the staff of the hospital or the patient's family and friends? These attitudes would seem strange in many cultures where the family's involvement in healing is strongly supported and viewed as essential to the process.

Addressing the Needs of Families

There are many reasons to address the needs of family members and involve them in the care of the patient. Again, *Through the Patient's Eyes* (Gerteis, Edgman-Levitan, Daley, and Delbanco, 1993) reminds us that

- Patients depend on their family to advocate for them.

- Patients usually need and want family members to be involved in care and decision making.

- Families and friends take care of sick people.

- Sickness affects the whole family.

- Families influence health behavior, health status and clinical outcomes, and patterns of service use.

- The family is a present client and a future customer.

The patient safety movement has also emphasized the importance of involving family members and friends in the quest to reduce medical errors. They are often the eyes and ears of the patient, and if encouraged, they will let the staff know when they see problems.

At one Planetree hospital, this point was clearly illustrated when a family member averted a potentially fatal medication error. Inadvertently, a patient's heparin lock was flushed with insulin. The patient's wife noticed a significant change in her husband's condition and notified the nurse. Valuing family involvement, the staff was able to quickly identify the problem and take immediate action to reverse the situation. Had the family not been involved, this incident might have had a far different outcome.

When patients are discharged, the family members take over as the primary caregivers, and they need the information and resources to do this effectively. They need to know what danger signs to watch for, who to call if there is a question, what to do in case of emergency, and how to handle treatments, dressing changes, medications, and numerous details necessary to help someone recover. Family members have an enormous amount of influence over how their loved one adjusts to and manages chronic conditions. Family members often control the eating habits of a person with chronic conditions, ensure that medications are taken correctly, and support or impede other rehabilitative activities and therapies.

Sickness, whether acute or chronic, affects the entire family. Family members and friends need information and emotional support to handle the impact of illness, just as the patient does. In

Grace and Grit (1991), Ken Wilber describes his experiences as a support person to his wife in her struggle against breast cancer. He shares the perspective of a friend, Vicky Wells, who had been a support person both for a sick family member and for Treya, Ken's wife. She says,

> I've been in both worlds—I've had cancer and I've been a support person for Treya and others. And I would have to say it is much harder being a support person. Because, at least for me, when I was dealing with my own cancer, there were lots of moments of sheer beauty and clarity and grace and reordering of priorities in life, and a reappreciation of the beauty of life. And I think that as a support person, that's really hard to find. The cancer person has no choice but to stay with it, but the support person has to choose to hang in there all the time. And it was real hard for me, as a support person[,] to get over the sadness, or get over the feeling of walking on eggshells around the person, or living with their treatment choices. What should I do and how should I support her? And should I be honest about what I really feel? It's an emotional roller coaster for the support person.

Family members can only speculate about the true experience of illness. Sometimes, imagining the impact of an illness is worse than the reality.

From a marketing perspective, the family members and friends are the hospital's next patients, *if* they like what they see and experience. With the fierce competition for survival in the health care industry, family members and friends should be treated as valued customers. In addition to the problems that families have with their involvement in the patient's care, they are very aware of aspects that the patient never sees. They know the effort involved in ensuring that their loved one receives good care. They know whether staff members are forthcoming with the information and support they need. Family members overhear staff conversations and they observe activities as they sit in waiting rooms or stroll the halls, which the patient never does. In the absence of publicly reported quality information, when deciding where to go for care, 70 percent of Americans have said that they would rely on the opinions of family members and friends as the most trusted source of information about a hospital, doctor, or health plan (Kaiser Family Foundation and Agency for Healthcare Research and Quality, 2000).

Strategies for Involving Families and Friends

The problems health care organizations have in addressing the needs of families stem from many sources—the way care is organized, the training and socialization of health care professionals, and the paternalistic culture that still reigns in many health care organizations. The implementation of new programs or approaches must acknowledge these factors to overcome the normal resistance most people have to changing "standard operating procedures."

Planetree Programs for Family Involvement

Planetree affiliates have developed and used a variety of effective strategies for involving the patient's social support network in hospital settings, including

- Care partner programs
- Birth partners
- Unrestricted visitation
- Collaborative care conferences
- Sharing clinical guidelines with family members
- Family spaces
- Pet visitation

Care Partner Programs

Many Planetree hospitals have implemented a simple program called Care Partners, which has become one of the best improvement strategies for involving and supporting family members and friends. This program can be adapted to many different settings, such as day surgery, emergency departments, or specialized testing settings.

When patients are admitted to the hospital or as part of the preadmission workup, they are asked to identify a family member or friend who will be their primary caregiver or support person. This care partner is usually a spouse or close relative, but he or she can be a friend or even someone hired to help. Care partners are identified by name in the chart and given buttons or nametags, making it easy for hospital staff members to identify them. With information and training, they are encouraged to assist with care and to enhance communication with the health care team.

Care partners are supported in a variety of ways to help them care for the patient. At some Planetree hospitals, they are served meals along with the patient or they are given discounted meal tickets for the cafeteria. In many facilities, they can stay in the room with the patient twenty-four hours a day if they choose to. They are also given other sources of support to encourage their involvement, such as discounted parking and discounted hotel rooms.

Care partners participate to the extent that they and the patient are comfortable. Many care partners use the opportunity to learn and practice the caregiving skills that may be needed when the patient goes home. Giving tube feedings, dressing changes, and helping to position patients are among the many skills that care partners learn. Those who are not interested in providing hands-on care may help support the patient emotionally, bringing in favorite music or cooking a special meal.

Perhaps the most meaningful part of the program is that care partners are encouraged to be active participants in the care process. They are advised to speak up with their questions and to challenge

anything that doesn't seem right, such as unexpected tests or procedures, unexplained medications, or adverse reactions. According
to Donna Taylor, care partner coordinator at Highline Community
Hospital in Burien, Washington, "They are respected and vital partners in the care of the patient and work closely with the staff to
ensure quality care. Once a care partner program is established, most
staff nurses find these family caregivers to be a valuable and time-
saving asset in addressing the patient's needs."

Birth Partners

Hudson River Healthcare in Peekskill, New York, a network of ten
federally funded health centers focusing on the underserved, created
the Planetree Maternal Care Partner Program. This award-winning
prenatal education and incentive program works to improve birth outcomes and the health of postpartum women and newborns. The care
partner may be a family member, a friend, or an AmeriCorp/Vista volunteer who, after completing an intensive training program, provides
support throughout the prenatal and postpartum period. Care partners
are from the same community as the participants in the program and
are able to offer education and support in a culturally familiar manner.

In the first year, 98 percent of those enrolled in the program
maintained their regularly scheduled prenatal and postpartum
appointments. As a result of the program, an average estimated savings of $150,000 is achieved for each infant who is not born with a
low birth weight.

Unrestricted Visitation

Whereas many hospitals have relaxed their visiting policies, most
Planetree hospitals have eliminated visiting restrictions altogether,
including in critical care areas. Griffin Hospital created a new configuration for its intensive care unit, giving families twenty-four-
hour access to the patient.

The emergency department is another area that has typically
restricted family visitation, even though, from the family's perspective,

it is often more important to be involved and present in an emergency room than in other less critical situations. Research has shown that families want to be with their loved ones in emergency rooms, even during such invasive procedures as cardiopulmonary resuscitation. A recent study found that the family benefited from being present and suffered no ill effects from having witnessed these events. Being present during crisis situations alleviates the family's anxiety and fear and helps with the process of bereavement (Meyers and others, 2000).

The emergency department at Alegent Health System's Bergan Mercy Medical Center in Omaha, Nebraska, has a policy of never separating the patient from the family. There is no limitation on how many family members may be present. According to Kevin Schwedhelm, the department's director, family members don't need to be "brought into the room" during code situations, because "they are already there." He believes that this policy contributes to their high patient satisfaction and limits the department's liability because it reduces the family's anger and, in the event the patient's death, reassures them that everything possible was done for the patient.

Many years ago, an emergency room the Picker Institute was working with was trying to convince the staff to let family members stay with acute myocardial infarction patients and other patients with serious conditions. The nurses were the most resistant, convinced that families would get in the way. The policy was changed but only after a hard lesson. One evening, a man was brought in from his house in a serious condition: he had a rapidly progressing heart attack. His teenage son insisted on being allowed to see him but the staff refused. The son was so agitated that security had to be called and the situation escalated into a confrontation with the family. Meanwhile, the father coded and died. In the aftermath, the staff learned that the father had collapsed in the midst of an argument with his son and the son wanted to tell his father he was sorry. It never happened. A simple act of kindness, letting the son in to apologize to his father, would have perhaps given the young man a sense of peace and resolution in the midst of his grief, rather than undying hatred for a cold and insensitive adherence to "hospital policy."

Collaborative Care Conferences

The collaborative care conference (described in greater detail in Chapter Two) brings together the physician, the nurse, the patient, and the family within the first twenty-four hours of admission, to clarify goals and expectations of the treatment plan and to discuss discharge planning. The conference encourages patient and family participation in decisions regarding care, and it identifies the family's needs so that they can be addressed before discharge.

Sharing Clinical Guidelines with Family Members

Sharing clinical guidelines or pathways with the family and patient is another powerful family and patient-centered improvement strategy. This one act addresses almost every dimension of patient- and family-centered care: respect, family involvement, information and education, coordination of care, and emotional support and transition. It has the added advantage of improving employee satisfaction after some predictable initial resistance. Ideally, these guidelines are provided to patients and families upon admission or when they come in for preadmission workups. Family members will see what the expected length of stay is and can immediately start preparing for the patient's discharge. Doctors sometimes fail to inform patients in advance of what the expected length of stay is. This can be a source of frustration when the family finds out that the patient will be discharged in three days when they were prepared for a ten-day stay. Informing family members of the expected length of stay is an excellent example of "anticipatory guidance" for them.

When families use guidelines to monitor the clinical course, they are often the first to identify problems. The guidelines often trigger questions and discussion that can help patients and their families become better managers of long-term chronic problems. When encountering initial resistance from staff members in the use of such guidelines, it is helpful to identify a physician who is willing to pilot the *patient pathways* with a few patients. Clinical staff members usually find that families, once thought of as difficult, are now helpful participants. The families now have clear expectations of the clinical encounter, are informed and knowledgeable, are ready to go home at the time of discharge, and feel that they have been respected partners in the care process.

Griffin Hospital in Derby, Connecticut, has developed a series of patient pathways for over fifteen common diagnoses. These are provided to patients and their families during the collaborative care conference.

Family Spaces

Typical hospital architecture often fails to take into account the involvement of the family. A sparsely furnished waiting room may be the only space available for families, friends, and visitors. If families are to be actively involved in the patients' care, then adequate and useful spaces need to be incorporated into the design. Kitchens enable families to prepare the patient's favorite food or make a meal for themselves. Libraries and lounges offer alternative spaces for a family when the patient needs privacy or is sleeping. Healing gardens and chapels can provide a spiritual refuge.

Planetree hospitals with private rooms often include a day bed or a sleeper chair in each room for overnight accommodations. Both Delano Regional Medical Center in Delano, California, and Windber Medical Center in Windber, Pennsylvania, included murphy beds in the renovation of medical and surgical units. Some hospitals also provide more extensive family accommodations elsewhere in the hospital. Aurora BayCare in Green Bay, Wisconsin, designed its new facility with twenty-two hotel-like rooms, equipped with refrigerators and seating areas. These rooms are available to families for a modest fee. Stratton VA Medical Center renovated a unit no longer being used for patient rooms to create hotel-like accommodations, called "the Hop-Tel." The Stratton campus also includes the Fisher House, which provides families with kitchen and laundry facilities.

Pet Visitation

For some patients, the support network extends beyond their human family and friends, to include companion animals. These "family members" can provide comfort and reassurance to patients, whether they are hospitalized briefly or for extended periods. In addition to traditional pet therapy, some Planetree affiliates have instituted programs that enable visits from the patients' own pets, often referred to as "POPs" programs. Both Longmont United Hospital in Longmont, Connecticut, and Avery Health Care System in Avery, North Carolina, use a simple checklist to ensure that the animal is kept on a leash when not in the patient's room and has the necessary vaccinations.

Family Involvement with Chronic Illness

Family members and other care partners are an integral part of care for patients with chronic illness. They influence a patient's health behavior, health status, and adherence to medical regimens (Speice and others, 2000). Studies have shown that support from friends and family is associated with improvement in the patient's functional status (Tsouna-Hadjus, Vemmos, Zakapoulos, and Stamatelopoulos, 2000), can reduce the patient's distress (Crystal and Kersting, 1998), and ease the adaptation to chronic impairment (Reinhardt, 1996).

Chronic illness affects 44 percent of the U.S. population, and of those with a chronic illness, more than half have two or more conditions (Committee on Quality of Health Care in America, 2001). Chronic illness places a significant burden on patients as well as on their families. Practitioners must be prepared to address both the physical and the psychological aspects of caring for patients with a chronic condition. The emotional reaction to the diagnosis of chronic illness can be more overwhelming than coping with symptoms of the illness (Lewis, 1998). Patients often experience anger, depression, and hopelessness, while their families deal with pervasive sadness, resentment, guilt, and loss (White and Grenyer, 1999). Individuals who cannot manage their illness will stop working earlier and will use more health care resources (Bogle, Percy, and Morrison, 1999). The demographics of our aging population and an increase in chronic conditions with shortened hospitalizations create a challenge for health care professionals, but they also offer an opportunity for partnership with family and friends in caring for patients with chronic health problems.

Recognizing this, health care institutions are experimenting with ways to involve family and friends in the care of a patient. One model that has been adopted widely is the cooperative care model. Most cooperative care programs emphasize patient and family education and responsibility in the hospital setting. When admitted, patients are accompanied by a care partner, who serves as a supportive companion and the "eyes and ears" for the medical staff. Other programs involve care partners in discharge preparation, education about home care, and legal and financial planning.

The Stanford Chronic Disease Self-Management Program

Professionals at the Stanford University School of Medicine in California noted that arthritis patients often had two or more chronic conditions and as a result were overwhelmed with information about disease management. Researchers developed and evaluated community-based self-management programs for people with multiple chronic health problems.

The Chronic Disease Self-Management Program is a six-week workshop held in community settings and facilitated by two trained peer leaders, one or both of whom have chronic diseases. Friends, partners, and spouses are encouraged to attend. The course covers

- Techniques to deal with frustration, fatigue, pain, and isolation

- Problem solving and decision making

- Appropriate exercise for maintaining and improving strength, flexibility, and endurance

- Appropriate use of medications

- Communicating effectively with family, friends, and health professionals

- Nutrition

- How to evaluate new treatments

Over twelve hundred people with heart disease, lung disease, stroke, and arthritis have participated in the course. At six months, the participants had increased their exercise, improved communication with their doctors, had fewer hospitalizations, felt less fatigued, had less pain, and were more socially active. At three years, participants continued to report greater confidence, less health distress, and fewer visits to physicians, even though their disability had increased (Lorig and others, 2001).

Additional Family Involvement Strategies

Patient Family Advisory Councils

One of the most effective strategies for involving families and patients in the design of care is to create patient-family advisory councils (Webster and Johnson, 2000). These councils, first designed and advanced by the Institute for Family-Centered Care in Bethesda, Maryland, invite patients and families who represent the constituencies served by the organization to become members of a council that meets regularly with senior hospital leaders. They serve as "listening posts" for the staff and provide a structure and process for ongoing dialogue and creative problem solving between the organization and its patients and families. The councils can play many roles, but they do not function as boards; nor do they have fiduciary responsibility for the organization. It is important to involve both families and patients, because they see different things and they each have an important perspective to consider.

Council responsibilities may include

- Prior program development, implementation, and evaluation

- Planning for major renovation or the design of a new building or services

- Staff selection and training

- Marketing hospital services

- Participation in staff orientation and in-service training programs

- Program development, implementation, and evaluation

- Marketing issues

These councils help overcome a common problem that most organizations face when they begin to develop patient- and family-centered processes: they do not have the direct experience of illness or the health care system.

Health care professionals often approach the design process from their own perspective, not the patients' or families'. Improvement committees with the best of intentions may disagree about who understands the needs of the patient and his or her family best. Patients and their family members rarely understand professional turf boundaries. Their suggestions are usually inexpensive, straightforward, and easy to implement, because they are not bound by the usual rules and sensitivities.

In general, when starting a patient family advisory council, it is best to start with members who are recommended by the staff—

people who can listen and respect different opinions. They should be supportive of the institution's mission as well as constructive with their input. They also need to be comfortable speaking to groups and in front of professionals. Most councils start off with one-year terms for all the members, to allow for graceful departures for members who are not well suited for the council.

The manual created by the Institute for Family-Centered Care in Bethesda, Maryland, *Developing and Sustaining a Patient and Family Advisory Council* (Webster and Johnson, 2000), is an excellent resource for organizations ready to establish these councils.

Walkthroughs

Performing a walkthrough is an effective way of re-creating for the staff the emotional and physical experiences of being a patient or a patient's family member. In addition to the Planetree staff retreat exercises described in Chapter One, walkthroughs provide a different perspective and bring to light rules and procedures that may have outlived their usefulness. This method of observation was developed by David Gustafson at the University of Wisconsin in Madison and was adapted by the Picker Institute to incorporate the staff perspective.

During a walkthrough, one staff member plays the role of the patient and another accompanies the patient as the family member. They go through a service or procedure or hospitalization exactly as a patient and his or her family members do. They do everything patients and families are asked to do, and they abide by the same rules. They do this openly, not as a mystery patient, and throughout the process they ask staff members a series of questions to encourage reflection on the processes or systems of care and to identify improvement opportunities. Notes are taken that document what they see and how they feel going through the walkthrough. These are then shared with the leaders of the organization, as well as with quality improvement teams, to help develop improvement plans. For many who do this, it is the first time they have ever entered their emergency rooms, operating rooms, or even clinics as patients.

Summary

For involving families and friends in the patient's care, there is one simple guideline that can be followed for all interactions and policies: never separate family members and friends from the patient— unless the patient requests it. Healing and recovery are enhanced by the love and support offered by a patient's community of family and friends. If we learn to incorporate that support, we will no longer be at odds with those who love and know the patient best. Family members are, and will be after the discharge, significant caregivers for the patient, and they need to be prepared for the new challenges to be faced.

References

Bogle, N., Percy, M., and Morrison, W. "Will I Make It Through This Choppy Water? A Psychological Characteristic as a Predeterminant Factor to Coping with Multiple Sclerosis." *Axone*, 1999, *20*(3), 3–66.

Botelho, R. J., Lue, B. H., and Fiscella, K. "Family Involvement in Routine Health Care: A Survey of Patients' Behaviors and Preferences." *Journal of Family Practice*, 1996, *42*(6), 572–576.

Committee on Quality of Health Care in America, Institute of Medicine. *Crossing the Quality Chasm: A New Health System for the Twenty-First Century*. Washington, D.C.: National Academies Press, 2001.

Crystal, S., and Kersting, R. C. "Stress, Social Support and Distress in a Statewide Population of Persons with AIDS in New Jersey." *Social Work Health Care*, 1998, *28*(1), 1–60.

Ellers, B. "Involving and Supporting Family and Friends." In M. Gerteis, S. Edgman-Levitan, J. Daley, and T. Delbanco (eds.), *Through the Patient's Eyes: Understanding and Promoting Patient-Centered Care*. San Francisco: Jossey-Bass, 1993.

Gerteis, M., Edgman-Levitan, S., Daley, J., and Delbanco, T. (eds.). *Through the Patient's Eyes: Understanding and Promoting Patient-Centered Care*. San Francisco, Jossey-Bass, 1993.

Kaiser Family Foundation and Agency for Healthcare Research and Quality. *Americans as Health Care Consumers: An Update on the Role of Quality Information*. Washington, D.C.: Kaiser Family Foundation and Agency for Healthcare Research and Quality, 2000.

Lewis, K. S. "Emotional Adjustment to a Chronic Illness." *Lippincott's Primary Care Practitioner,* 1998, *2*(1), 38–51.

Lorig, K., and others. "Chronic Disease Self-Management Program: Two-Year Health Status and Health Care Utilization Outcomes." *Medical Care,* 2001, *39*(11), 1217–1223.

Meyers, T., and others. "Original Research: Family Presence During Invasive Procedures and Resuscitation." *American Journal of Nursing,* 2000, *100*(2), 32.

Reinhardt, J. P. "The Importance of Friendship and Family Support in the Adaptation to Chronic Vision Impairment." *The Journals of Gerontology, Series B: Psychological Sciences,* 1996, *51*(5), 268–278.

Speice, J., and others. "Involving Family Members in Cancer Care: Focus Group Considerations of Patients and Oncological Providers." *Psychooncology,* 2000, *9*(2), 101–112.

Tsouna-Hadjus, E., Vemmos, K. N., Zakapoulos, N., and Stamatelopoulos, S. "First Stroke Recovery Process: The Role of Family Social Support." *Archives of Physical Medicine Rehabilitation,* 2000, *81*(7), 881–887.

vom Eigen, K. A., and others. "Carepartner Experiences with Hospital Care." *Medical Care,* 1999, *37*(1), 33–38.

Webster, P. D., and Johnson, B. *Developing and Sustaining a Patient and Family Advisory Council.* Bethesda, Md.: Institute for Family-Centered Care, 2000.

White, Y., and Grenyer, B. F. "The Biopsychosocial Impact of End-Stage Renal Disease: The Experience of Dialysis Patients and Their Partners." *Journal of Advanced Nursing,* 1999, *30*(6), 1312–1320.

Wilber, K. *Grace and Grit: Spirituality and Healing in the Life and Death of Treya Killam Wilber.* Boston: Shambhala, 1991.

4

Nutrition

The Nurturing Aspects of Food

Kathy Reinke and Carol Ryczek

Hippocrates, whose healing legacy is so fundamental to the Planetree philosophy, made a connection between food and health over two thousand years ago, when he advised, "Let food be your medicine." Food, of course, is an integral part of health. In addition to its nourishing aspects, food has the power to comfort and heal—or cause anxiety and aversion. Eating can be a powerful symbol of nurturing, love, and celebration. But which foods fit in the overall healing experience? How can they be incorporated into food service plans that work for the individual as well as for the hospital? Health care facilities have a responsibility to provide food that is both nurturing and nourishing, and to empower individuals to achieve healthful eating habits in their daily lives.

Hospitals struggle with the logistics of feeding patients in an environment of ever-changing diet orders, room changes, therapeutic restrictions, and a fluctuating census. Several times a day, the food service department faces the challenge of planning and preparing a menu of foods to meet a variety of nutritional needs, observing all health and food safety codes, delivering meals in a timely manner to patients in rooms all over the hospital, and keeping hot foods hot and cold foods cold. Add to that the increasing pressure that food service programs face in controlling cost and in doing more with fewer staff members. It is no mystery that many hospital dietary departments adopt the attitude, "There—you're fed. Good enough."

But at what expense? For the public, hospital food has joined the undistinguished company of school lunches and airline food as meals of last resort. At the very least, many hospital kitchens seem to have discarded the notion that eating should be a pleasurable experience. Greeting card manufacturer Hallmark, Inc., has used humor about hospital food on many get-well cards—for example, "This card is made of a special substance that actually tastes better than hospital food!" Open the card and the message reads, "It's called cardboard!" Another sign that hospital food has permeated the culture as an icon of something distasteful is the punk rock band that calls itself Hospital Food, as it compares its disturbing sound to something deemed equally unpleasant (Hospital Food, 2002).

We know that uneaten food provides no nourishment. In 1974, Butterworth drew attention to "the skeleton in the hospital closet"—namely, mismanagement of patients' nutritional health. He found that many patients left the hospital more malnourished than when they entered. He then challenged institutions to make "relatively modest revisions of attitude, administrative effort, and financial support [that] could reverse this neglect and pay rich dividends" (Butterworth, 1974, p. 440). An enormous improvement has been seen since then, not only in patient monitoring and diagnosis, but in the delivery of nutrition support as well (Harkness, 2002). Thankfully, there is evidence that the likelihood of developing malnutrition during hospitalization has decreased in the past two decades (Blackburn, 1995). Adequate nutrition can be more easily assured with the availability of specialized enteral and parenteral formulations.

As the science of nutrition support has improved, the "soft" features of meal service have been pushed aside in many hospitals. Institutions seem to have forgotten that "food" and "service" are at the heart of food service. The Planetree model has long recognized the power of food to nourish body *and* soul. Common approaches shared by many Planetree health care facilities include locating homelike kitchens in patient care areas, providing "comfort foods"—those familiar foods that evoke a caring, pleasant feeling even before they are tasted—healthy choices and options, and a meal delivery system that is as homelike as possible. Providing nourishment is more than just providing the right number of calories; it is taking care that the appearance, presentation, aromas, flavors, delivery, and setting are optimal as well. Meals are often the highlight of the patient's day. They may provide a few minutes of pleasure in a stay otherwise interrupted by painful and unpleasant injections, procedures, and treatments.

There is no "cookbook" approach to developing a Planetree nutrition program. It does not require a specific menu or food delivery system. It will vary according to the size of the facility, the culture, the interaction of its disciplines, and the needs of its patients and community. It begins, as do so many aspects of Planetree, with assessing the needs of patients from their perspective. What nutritional resources do patients want? Are staff members empowered to make changes and improvements to enhance the patient's experience of nourishment while in the hospital?

Too often, food service staff members are not appreciated for the important role they play in the patients' overall experience. Patients may not be able to assess the skill of the surgeon in the operating room, or the nurse dispensing medication, but they can and do evaluate the meals set before them. Empowering food service staff members at all levels is critical to achieving and maintaining good results. Incorporating the Planetree philosophy into food service is not the job of one person or one department. It takes an integrated approach, budget consideration, and support by staff members in several key areas to make it work.

"Let staff know [that] they won't be punished for taking a risk" is an important message from Phyllis Stoneburner, vice-president of patient care services at Warren Memorial Hospital in Front Royal, Virginia. "You can 'what if?' things to death" (personal interview, Feb. 18, 2002). At Warren Memorial, a process improvement team, with representatives from housekeeping, dietary, nursing, and administration, met weekly for six months as they prepared to change their meal delivery system. They saw this as an opportunity for recognizing the value of food as a part of care and treatment, and for enhancing clinical outcomes.

Serving Patients: The Planetree Approach

Nutrition has always been viewed as one of the core components in the Planetree model of care. The original model site at Pacific Presbyterian Medical Center in San Francisco, California, added a kitchen to provide an area where patients' families could prepare their loved ones' favorite foods. In addition, a nutritionist was available to provide patients with individualized nutrition plans and to teach good nutrition through cooking demonstrations. The kitchen made food available twenty-four hours a day, and it became the meeting place of many of the patients' families.

The nutrition program must be structured to acknowledge that there is a person on the receiving end of the food line. Individuals come to a hospital with a lifetime of food preferences, eating experiences, and expectations. Their meal service should follow the same theme as other Planetree care: it should personalize, demystify, and humanize.

Prior to changing their meal selection system, dietary workers at Longmont United Hospital in Longmont, Colorado, observed that they were "too busy chasing paper to realize [that] there was a person attached to it." They have since implemented a room service–style menu, in which meal selections are taken by phone. Patients call the kitchen themselves, or a food service employee calls the patient. ("They love for us to call them.") The menu and special modifications are discussed, and opportunities for education by the dietitian arise. A patient on a low-salt diet who requests gravy will not be denied his or her choice. However, the discussion with the dietitian will include information on how to flavor gravy without salt (Sheila West, telephone interview, Mar. 12, 2002).

A study of current and future practices in hospital food service confirms that the environment is changing. Food service directors expect to serve meals to fewer inpatients, employ fewer staff members, have smaller expense budgets, and generate more revenue in the future (Silverman, 2002). Although there is no consensus as to how best to respond to these trends, one common issue identified was the need to intensify the focus on patient satisfaction—seeing the patient as our customer and exceeding service expectations (Lambert, 1999).

Personalized Service

As with many other aspects of health care, the key to improving patient nutrition and satisfaction is in providing more personalized service. Eating has long been a social activity that may become lost, as one lies isolated in a hospital bed. The staff at Warren Memorial found a way to increase social interaction with their in-room dining service. A dietary staff person comes into the patient's room a few minutes before mealtime to talk about the planned menu, ready to offer a substitution if it seems appropriate. As they talk, the bedside table is cleared of clutter, similar to what one might do to prepare the patient's kitchen table at home before mealtime. A place mat is set, a folded napkin placed to the side. The dinner plate arrives, freshly served up at the tray assembly area, located right on the nursing unit. Sending in the people who have helped prepare the meal provides ownership in the part they play in the patient's food service experience. The food service staff members hear comments directly from the patients.

The growing trend of room service menu programs in hospitals also speaks to the industry's attempt to improve patient satisfaction with food service (Robinson, 2000). A restaurant-style menu, with a variety of appealing choices, is available to patients to order what they want, when they want it. The loss of control that many patients experience during a hospitalization may cause great anxiety and frustration. Allowing them choices in eating returns some of that control. "Concurrent efforts to reduce costs and improve patient satisfaction and customer service have led many (Food Service Directors) to initiate 'point-of-service' meal delivery systems from their mobile carts over the last two years" (Lawn, 2002, p. 30).

Aurora Bay Care Hospital in Green Bay, Wisconsin, planned for a room service meal delivery system from its outset. The newly built facility includes a restaurant-style kitchen under the direction of a chef trained in the "hospitality" model.

A chef can be a welcome addition to the hospital environment, but some very basic menu systems can also yield consistently high patient satisfaction scores. At Shawano Medical Center in Shawano, Wisconsin, the patient meal service follows a one-week cycle of basic familiar comfort foods of the population it serves. Individualized care is provided by obtaining the patient's food preferences and dislikes and making modifications to his or her menu as needed. Most patients are not fussy. They are not on vacation; they have other priorities. Again, often it is just the fact that someone has asked them if they would like something special to eat (personalized attention) that means as much as the actual food provided. There is a list of alternative choices available to offer the patient, the most popular of which is chicken noodle soup. In fact, the long-held view of soup as a comfort food was reinforced when the emergency room staff of Shawano Medical Center in Shawano, Wisconsin, started a campaign to help reduce the amount of antibiotics prescribed for inappropriate (viral) illnesses. They created a "cold kit," which includes, among other things, a packet of tissues, an over-the-counter cough remedy, and a package of instant chicken soup. The message is that "while we can't provide a cure, we can offer comfort."

Hold the Institutional Look, Please

It is important to take a close look at how food is perceived from the patient's point of view. There are obvious quality markers: Did the patient get the correct food choice? Is the coffee hot? Is the milk cold? There are the more subtle perceptions of quality as well. How is the meal presented? Is it served in faded mugs and bowls? Does the china pattern complement the plate presentation? A colorful tray liner can provide color and brightness as the meal is placed in front of the patient. The cooks at Shawano Medical Center have chosen to forgo the standard four-ounce foam-packaged container of ice cream. Instead, they hand-scoop ice cream into raised glass stemware and drizzle it with chocolate syrup for a pleasing presentation. The consumption of milk and juice increased when cartons and aseptically sealed containers were replaced with drinking glasses. It appears that the familiarity of drinking beverages in the same type of dishware people use at home made a difference. Eliminating the barrier of trying to open super-sealed containers probably helped as well.

The process of eating involves many senses. When the plate cover is lifted from the tray, what is the first impression? It is hoped that it is not the distinct odor of cooked broccoli or fish, which even a hungry person may find offensive. What does the patient see? Is there an interesting mix of color, size, and texture of foods? Too often, a cluttered tray or portions that are too large can overwhelm a patient who is not feeling well and has a small appetite to start with.

The element of surprise can also enhance presentation. Include an appropriate garnish on the cook's production menu. Send a child's cereal in their favorite cartoon character bowl. Surprise patients with a fresh flower; it may be the only one some patients receive during their entire stay.

Special Diets

The food restrictions of special diets can make it a challenge to send a tray that looks appealing. One example is a traditional full-liquid diet, often used as a transition from a clear liquid diet (broth, some juice, gelatin) to a general diet. The traditional full-liquid diet allows foods of a "liquid nature," such as strained oatmeal, creamed soup, milk, or tomato juice. Shawano Medical Center staff members saw patients rejecting many of these items and often asking for items that were not allowed on the diet. A quality improvement team, with the input of the medical staff, developed an alternative diet to serve as the bridge to tolerating a general diet. The new diet, called "semi-liquid," includes all of the items commonly included, with the addition of some of the solid foods frequently requested by patients as they resume normal eating, such as crackers, toast, or mashed potatoes. Sending chicken noodle soup, as opposed to the strained cream of chicken soup specified on a full liquid diet, reflects the desire to incorporate the perceived comfort foods. The new semiliquid diet has been well received by patients, nurses, and physicians.

Planetree Pantries

The kitchen pantry area on a nursing unit can serve several functions. It may simply be the place where crackers and juice are kept for a between-meal snack or where extra jelly packets or tea bags might be found. In a Planetree hospital, the pantry is often expanded to provide a kitchen area and dining tables for patients and their families. Given the diversity of the American diet, cultural preferences of patients may be best met by providing an area where family members can prepare favorite foods for their loved ones. Just as the family kitchen tends to be where people congregate in their homes, so, too, can the Planetree pantry serve as a gathering place for patients and families, creating opportunities for spontaneous support groups during hospitalization. This is an area where volunteers and nutritionists can conduct food demonstrations and classes, providing nutrition information to help equip the patient with necessary skills for following a special diet at home. Volunteers may bake cookies, muffins, and breads, letting the fresh-baked aroma drift through the halls.

Not all Planetree pantries look alike. For some, a microwave, refrigerator, and disposable dishes may be sufficient. Others may have a fully equipped working kitchen, complete with stove, sink, dishwasher, cooking utensils, and china. A multidisciplinary team can explore and discuss possibilities that reflect the individual style and needs of the patient care unit. What is essential is a warm and inviting atmosphere to make patients and their families feel comfortable.

Keeping It Clean

Hospital safety, sanitation, and regulatory standards need to be addressed as the Planetree pantry is developed. Involving all appropriate staff members is necessary to be sure that there is a clear understanding of duties and responsibilities. Plant operations, for example, must be comfortable with the electrical equipment furnished on the pantry unit. Who cleans the refrigerator? Is it a dietary, nursing, or housekeeping assignment? Where are the cleanup supplies kept? Every hospital develops its own way of making sure that the critical elements necessary to ensure a clean and safe pantry are addressed. Some Planetree pantries may be equipped for dishwashing, whereas other hospitals send dirty dishes and utensils to the dietary kitchen for proper cleaning and sanitizing.

Likewise, food safety precautions cannot be overlooked. For the health and safety of everyone using the pantry, guidelines for use need to be clearly communicated. For example, guidelines would likely include directions for proper hand washing, information regarding labeling and storage of foods, and what restrictions may apply to pantry use. These may be reviewed with the patient and his or her family as part of the initial room orientation process. Stocking the pantry with single-service packaged food items provides less chance of contamination.

It is also important that staff members understand their responsibilities to make sure the pantry is functioning as intended. Planetree pantry guidelines should be included in the new employee orientation for the nursing and dietary staff. Any special dietary concerns of patients need to be considered, and, again, they should be clearly communicated to the patient and his or her family. This can provide some great teaching moments. For example, a nurse might say, "This fresh apple muffin you brought in from home looks great, Mrs. Smith. It might be just what your husband needs to perk up his appetite. If we omit the bread and applesauce from his dinner tray, the carbohydrate content will stay within the guidelines of his diabetic diet."

Individual nursing units may have their own criteria in deciding what foods to stock in their pantry, according to its intended use. Having a pantry is a special opportunity, and all involved need to do their part to make sure it is respected as such.

Hospital Cafeterias

The hospital cafeteria has often been relegated to the basement or an out-of-the-way corner of the hospital, seemingly as an after-thought for an ancillary activity. But if every employee is a care-giver, every part of the hospital can be designed to deliver care. In this context, the hospital cafeteria can play a role in community health and health education; it can provide a welcome refuge for patients and visitors and can contribute to employee satisfaction. With this in mind, many Planetree facilities have reshaped their cafeterias to reflect their new role, upgrading them with light, color, visibility, and food selections that are healthy and appealing. Many have a garden or patio. Windows and artwork provide an opportu-nity to "escape" visually. Patient rooms, which need to be shelter-ing and soothing, tend to be darker. The contrast of a sunny, bright cafeteria or café environment can be welcoming.

At Shawano Medical Center, a glass wall is all that separates the cafeteria from the main entrance corridor to the building. The cafete-ria, called the Riverside Café, opens out to a patio, fountain, and gar-den. The colors are soft, the chairs are wooden, and the food is good enough to attract regular nonpatient patrons from the community. As in many Planetree hospitals, coffee, tea, and broth are served free throughout the day to patients, visitors, and staff members. This ges-ture establishes a sense of hospitality that sets the tone for the visit, and costs are recouped in public relations and patient satisfaction dividends.

The cafeteria's placement at the entrance to Longmont United Hospital makes it a popular meeting place for community mem-bers. People who use the hospital's fitness area, located near the cafeteria, often stop in after an exercise class to have a snack or share free coffee.

At Aurora BayCare Medical Center's Greenbrier Café, tables and booths are scattered along a graceful curve. Large windows provide a view of the outdoors, even when Green Bay's northern climate keeps patrons from using the patio tables. A value-pricing system at Aurora BayCare is another expression of its Planetree philosophy. Visitors and staff members pay the same for each item, reflecting the idea that the staff works in partnership with, not separately from, the public they serve.

Nutrition Information

A hospital cafeteria can provide food for the mind as well as for the body and soul by incorporating a healthy eating philosophy into the menu choices. Shawano Medical Center's cafeteria is known in the community as a healthy place to eat. A salad bar is always available. Low- or no-fat condiments and low-fat milk products are always available. And while the menu may include some higher-fat entrees, low-fat, low-salt, fiber-rich, fruit-and-vegetable-intense meals are always an option. Shawano's Riverside Café also permits half-servings of entrees and charges for salad items by the ounce. Fresh fruit, juices, hot and cold vegetables, and raisins are available every day. In addition to promoting good eating habits for the staff, the focus on nutritious choices provides the community with fast food that isn't fat food. A policy that allows small, free-of-charge "tastes" has helped broaden the acceptance of unfamiliar foods. Couscous, a staple in many parts of the world, was rarely found on northern Wisconsin plates. Encouraging patrons to sample small portions enabled them to try new flavors. Couscous is now a regular menu item at the Riverside Café, and it is hoped that it will be in many area homes as well.

A Family Refuge

A well-designed hospital cafeteria creates a refuge for families to gather away from patient care areas. In many households, family discussions are held around the kitchen table, so some Planetree facilities invite families to use the cafeteria, help themselves to free coffee or tea, and re-create this intimate family space in the cafeteria.

The special burden on families of patients hospitalized for longer stays provided the impetus for Longmont United Hospital to add a pizza oven to its cafeteria. Sheila West, manager of nutritional services at Longmont Hospital, observed that families visiting long-term patients were finding the cost of so many cafeteria meals to be a burden. "It's a hardship for some people. I know it takes a financial bite," she said. "A pizza can feed a family a nutritious meal for an affordable price and still keep the food purchase within the hospital" (telephone interview, Mar. 12, 2002).

The Value of Staff Interactions

The comforting aspects of a shared meal begin with the cafeteria staff. Visitors often arrive anxious, worried, and lonely. Kind words from the person serving a meal can be as nourishing as the food. Visitors also find comfort in chatting with approachable staff members. They build relationships—some just for a few days—that make long- and short-term patrons feel like "regulars."

At many Planetree hospitals, there is no sign asking visitors to allow staff members to go first. This would be like posting a sign that says, "Our time is valuable, but yours isn't."

Staff members are trained to be sensitive to the special needs of the population they serve, ready to carry a tray for someone with a walker, or read a menu for a person with a bandage over one eye. Once a month, the Wolf River Area Stroke Club (a support group for stroke survivors and families) visits Shawano Medical Center for a meeting and meal. They meet there with the assurance that the staff will respond with sensitivity—helping when needed or standing back when appropriate.

In addition to the impression created by the staff, the care with which the facility is tended creates a lasting impression of the cleanliness of the hospital. A visitor who is waiting for a surgical patient can't assess the cleanliness of the surgical suite, but he can and does assess whether the dining and serving area looks clean.

Aroma Therapy

Shawano Medical Center's cooks do most of their baking in the hospital kitchen, where the ventilating system carries the cooking smells out of the building. However, each morning, the breakfast server makes small batches of cookies in an oven in the cafeteria. The smell of the cookies or freshly baked bread lingers in the main hallway; so as patients enter the building, they are pleasantly surprised with a homey aroma instead of the expected "hospital smell."

The "aroma therapy" of baking cookies or bread can be a marketing tool to draw customers into the cafeteria. Many patients and visitors will stop at the cafeteria on their way out because they've been enticed by the smells. ("That smells great. . . . Let's grab breakfast in the cafeteria on our way out.")

As aromatherapists know, there is a close connection between smell and memory. "The perceived intensity of the odorants depend not only on stimulus concentration but probably also on experience-dependent factors" (Distel and others, 1999, p. 191). For many people, the memory of a typical hospital includes a blend of smells from disinfectants, alcohol wipes, and soiled linen. By baking cookies in the cafeteria, the unpleasant odors that most people associate with health care are replaced by something more familiar. Every building, every business, every home has a scent. Although staff members may no longer notice these smells, patients and visitors will be aware of some kind of odor as they walk in. It is safe to assume that the public would rather smell chocolate chip cookies than Betadine wash.

Warren Memorial Hospital recognized the strong associations created by smells. On Thanksgiving Day, volunteers cooked turkeys in the hospital's Planetree pantries, encouraging the aroma of a festive meal to drift throughout the building. Even patients who could not eat the turkey enjoyed the smell. Rather than feeling deprived, patients reported being able to smell the meal as it cooked, just as they would have at home, which made them feel a part of the holiday.

Community Nutrition Education

With a commitment to patient empowerment, Planetree hospitals provide patients with the education they need to make informed decisions about their care and their health. Dietitians, like other clinicians, encounter barriers to providing meaningful education in a hospital setting. Patients can be overwhelmed by the need to make changes in their diet, and they can have trouble translating the information into practical improvements in their eating habits. Nutrition education competes with medications, activity restrictions, and other follow-up instructions, and it may not be presented to patients until the day of discharge. Even information that is presented at more teachable moments during the course of the stay may not be understood clearly enough to be implemented upon returning home. The hospital's mission to improve community health adds the responsibility of providing lifestyle education not only to patients as they are discharged but to the wider population as well. Community education and outreach are ways to meet these educational needs. Community education is also a response to the public demand for diet and nutrition information.

"Nutrition and You: Trends 2000," an American Dietetic Association public opinion survey (Public Relations Team, 2000), reported that 85 percent of the people surveyed said that diet and nutrition issues are important to them personally. To obtain information, over 90 percent looked to nutritionists and physicians. Clearly, the public is hungry for information and look to the medical community as a trusted source.

Community Classes

The first component of many community outreach programs is a series of classes. Unfortunately, many hospitals find that attendance at these programs, however well-meaning and informative, is minimal at best. At Shawano Medical Center, the Main Course program was created to make nutrition education appealing by eliminating the barriers to attendance, and Main Course has succeeded by tailoring its program to the demands of a busy adult audience instead of to the convenience of the presenters. Monthly classes are held at several different times during the day. Classes are an hour long or less, include food samples, and cover topics such as "Nutrition on the Run," interspersed with information on traditional low-salt, low-fat diet presentations. Classes deliver clear, simple messages and focus on practical applications of nutrition theory rather than on the statistical basis for those choices (Patterson and others, 2001). A yearly schedule is publicized so that participants can select the topics that are most meaningful to them. Main Course is billed as "Nutrition Information Served the Way You Like It," and past participants in cardiac rehabilitation and nutrition counseling sessions have found the series helpful in that it provides ongoing support of their healthier eating style.

Heart Disease Reversal Programs

Many community programs provide small, sequential steps for enhancing the community's nutritional health and literacy. But for some people, this approach has proven to be "too little, too late." Windber Medical Center in Windber, Pennsylvania, approached health and nutrition education not as incremental change but as a complete change of lifestyle. Windber adopted the Dean Ornish Program for Reversing Heart Disease in January 2000, after Nick Jacobs, Windber's CEO, was served a typical breakfast of bacon and eggs while recovering from heart surgery (Jacobs, 2002).

In Windber's implementation of the Ornish program, food is not merely provided by the hospital but is viewed as a fundamental component of the healing process. The program includes a low-fat, vegetarian nutrition plan, stress management techniques, regular exercise, and group support. The benefits of the strict regime are improved blood flow through the heart, reduction in chest pain, and improvement in the quality of life, which includes more mobility and stamina. Although aimed at individual heart disease patients, the program is structured so that patients can take the concepts and diets with them into everyday life, outside the hospital setting (Ornish and others, 1998).

Potential participants are screened to make sure they are ready to follow the strict program guidelines; at Windber, 70 to 80 percent of the applicants make the commitment. Patients who are not good candidates for the Ornish program are included in the hospital's regular cardiac rehabilitation program.

The success of Windber's Ornish program (132 graduates in two years) is a testament to the hospital's commitment to the program. The facility that houses the program is attached to the hospital and boasts a 12,300-square-foot fitness, pool, and therapy area, an indoor walking track, a demonstration kitchen, classrooms for yoga, and meeting rooms for group discussions. It also houses the Dean Ornish Prostate Cancer Reversal Research Program, a cooperative study being done in conjunction with the Walter Reed Medical Center in Fairfax, Virginia, investigating molecular level changes.

Windber's gym is used by staff members as well as by community members, and it has become a social hub. Ornish participants now ask area restaurants to alter entrees to accommodate their low-fat cooking style. Ornish-compatible food selections are available at each meal in the hospital cafeteria. Participants and program graduates form a "self-directed community" and share recipes, potluck meals, and encouragement.

Food and Healing

It is ironic that one of the most fundamental of human needs has been considered the domain of an "ancillary department" in hospitals— a service for the structure of the institution rather than for the healing of patients. The Planetree adage that "everyone is a caregiver" is an apt reminder that every aspect of a patient's stay can contribute to his or her healing. Patients already know the importance of food. As hospitals explore the role that food can play, they will continue to discover ways to make nutrition an integral part of patient care and community health. Bringing a sense of community and caring to the hospital experience is a contribution well suited to nutrition services. Using the inherent symbolism of food to nurture, nourish, and comfort the body, mind, and spirit is an opportunity that exists in virtually all organizational settings. Recognizing the valuable role that dietary staff members can play in optimizing this opportunity, and engaging them in enhancing the patient's experience, is key to changing attitudes toward hospital food.

References

Blackburn, G. L., and Ahman, A. "Skeleton in the Hospital Closet—Then and Now." *Nutrition (Supplement)*, 1995, *11* (supp. 2), 193–195.

Butterworth, E., Jr. "The Skeleton in the Hospital Closet." *Nutrition Today*, 1974, 436–440.

Distel, H., and others. "Perception of Everyday Odors—Correlation Between Intensity, Familiarity and Strength of Hedonic Judgement." *Chemical Senses*, 1999, *24*, 191–199.

Harkness, L. "The History of Enteral Nutrition Therapy: From Raw Eggs and Nasal Tubes to Purified Amino Acids and Early Postoperative Jejunal Delivery." *Journal of the American Dietetic Association*, Mar. 2002, *102*, 399–404.

Hospital Food. "Hospital Food." Punk band Web site: [http://www.hospitalfood.net/main.htm]. Apr. 5, 2002.

Jacobs, F. N. Interview in *PlaneTalk*. Derby, Conn.: Planetree, Mar. 2002, p. 3.

Lambert, L. G., Boudreaux, J., Conklin, M., and Yadrick, K. "Are New Meal Distribution Systems Worth the Effort for Improving Patient Satisfaction with Foodservice?" *Journal of the American Dietetic Association*, 1999, 99(9), 1112–1114.

Lawn, J. "2002: A Cross-Segment Business Forecast." *Food Management*, Feb. 2002, pp. 16–30.

Ornish, D., and others. "Intensive Lifestyle Changes for Reversal of Coronary Heart Disease." *Journal of the American Medical Association*, 1998, *280*, 2001–2007.

Patterson, R. E., and others. "Is There a Consumer Backlash Against the Diet and Health Message?" *Journal of the American Dietetic Association*, 2001, *101*, 37–41.

Public Relations Team. "Nutrition and You: Trends 2000." *Journal of the American Dietetic Association*, 2000, *100*(6), 626–627.

Robinson, N. "Room Service: Another Success Story in the Making." *Health Care Food and Nutrition Focus*, 2000, *16*(7), 1, 3–5.

Silverman, M. R. "Current and Future Practices in Hospital Foodservice." *Journal of the American Dietetic Association*, Apr. 5, 2002. [http://findarticles.com/cf].

5

Spirituality

Inner Resources for Healing

George Handzo and Jo Clare Wilson

There has been a resurgence over the past ten years in the overall arena of spirituality. It is the subject of an array of best-selling books and magazines as well as popular television programs. It is often employed in the business world as companies look at benefits to the bottom line when employees' spiritual needs are met. Nowhere has this resurgence been addressed more rigorously in recent years than in health care. The world of medicine is making monumental efforts to address spiritual needs as a powerful ally of healing. In the last decade, interest in and research focused on spirituality and health has increased significantly. The number of articles, books, and conferences dedicated to studying the effects of spiritual practice on health and healing are overwhelming. The array of publications regarding spirituality within the context of health range from the research-oriented *Science and Theology* to a popular magazine entitled *Spirituality and Health*. The latter offers articles about a variety of spiritual practices, such as prayer, meditation, and yoga, whereas *Science and Theology* examines neurons in the brain for proof of the existence of God.

There is also an increase in the number of medical schools teaching classes focused on spirituality and the care of patients. As early as the 1980s, there was heightened interest in teaching physicians a more sensitive and caring style in their relationships with patients.

Doctors were encouraged to see the patient as more than a disease and to consider the whole person. There was renewed energy for patients to be more involved and participatory in their health care. These influences worked toward the growing view that science and medicine had overlooked the once accepted reality of the interrelatedness of mind, body, and spirit. As a factor in the equation, spirituality began to be taken more seriously within the healing process.

Hospital chaplains have always nurtured the spiritual link in health care. Many, in fact, are professionally trained in clinical pastoral care. But hospital chaplaincy has often viewed this as a function of religion. Yet most chaplains work with all patients, regardless of "religious affiliation," and the focus of the pastoral care is to understand the patient's concerns about making meaning out of what is happening to him or her in the midst of his or her illness, surgery, and healing.

Religion and Medicine: A Historical Review

Throughout much of human history and in many places in the world today, religion and medicine are joined. In many cultures, one individual is responsible for healing the body, mind, and spirit. The person is viewed as a whole. The advent of science brought the separation of those who cared for the body and the mind from those who cared for the spirit. Some scientists believed that religious belief and practice did not contribute to physical or psychic healing. Because the influence of religion on healing could not be proved by scientific standards, many medical practitioners believed that it therefore had no place in the treatment of disease.

Some members of the clergy and other religious leaders, in turn, believed that to be scientific was to be antireligious. They did not seek to be integrated into the medical treatment team. And some religious professionals held the belief that leaders from the patient's own faith group knew what would benefit the patient. There was little consideration given to the particular needs of the individual or to the possibility that the patient's beliefs might not conform to the traditional beliefs of that particular faith group.

In the early twentieth century, the awareness began to develop that the role of religion in any given person's life was quite individualistic. It became more apparent that religious belief and practice played an important role in how people dealt with suffering, but what that role was for any individual could not be predicted by simply finding out what faith group the person identified with. Furthermore, patients derived more benefit from their religious resources if they were able to identify the benefits on their own rather than being told what to believe or what rituals to practice.

Training programs began to develop in which members of the clergy are taught to elicit and listen to the stories and feelings of the patient or the patient's family members. The center of the pastoral care became relationship building and letting the patient direct the interaction. Pastoral caregivers were trained to minister to patients from any religious background and to structure their interventions to meet individual needs. They also saw themselves as intentional bridges between the science of medicine and the spirituality of religion. This style lends itself to integration with the medical treatment team and a return to a holistic treatment philosophy.

In recent years, two major developments have broadened the practice and influence of pastoral care. First, it became more widely recognized that the issues pastoral caregivers were dealing with often went beyond religious belief and practice. Basic human needs, such as finding meaning and sustaining hope, could be dealt with in religious terms but often fell into a broader realm of experience that became known as spiritual. Some people are officially religious, but it seems that most people have a sense of spirituality that can help them cope with suffering.

Second, cultural trends have helped to expand the focus of medical care to include not only physical symptoms but also other factors that may influence health. Along with social and psychological factors, spiritual and religious practices are being recognized as aspects in the treatment of any patient. Pastoral care is increasingly known as spiritual care and continues to become integrated into the practice of all members of the treatment team, often with the pastoral caregiver serving as the specialist. This system parallels that used in acute care settings for the treatment of psychological problems. All members of the treatment team are responsible for being aware of the patient's psychological issues, but certain professionals (psychologists, psychiatrists, and social workers) bear primary responsibility for the treatment of these issues as the need arises.

Working Definitions of Spirituality

There is general acceptance that spirituality is a broad concept that is distinct from but similar to religion (Mueller and Plevak, 2001). Spirituality is thought to be the overall experiential and dynamic process of finding meaning and connectedness in life. In comparison, religion is one of the many ways in which a person may exercise or practice his or her spirituality.

Religion focuses on specific principles and doctrines formulated around a set of beliefs in a particular faith. Spirituality is a larger concept that may be defined and understood as the inner life, which enables us to make meaning and find value through connectedness to a transcendent whole and which fosters our self-understanding. The impact or result of maintaining a spiritual practice creates a sense of hope and purpose in one's existence.

Research has indicated a relationship between spirituality and health that is primarily positive. One of the ways to understand the effects of a spiritual practice on the healing process is to look at studies regarding the placebo effect. Studies done to determine what factors are in place when control groups are given a placebo with a positive outcome have shown that there are three important variables that effect healing. These are (1) a supportive and caring group to which a person maintains connection, (2) a sense of mastery and control over self (note that this is meant as mastery and control over not the disease but, rather, the response to the disease), and (3) the ability to make meaning out of the disease or illness (Siegel, 1984).

How Spirituality Works as an Inner Resource

For most of us, there is a commonsense understanding that these three factors would be of value in shaping how a person structures his or her *beliefs* about the healing process. To have supportive people around us, to feel that we have control, and to take a positive rather than negative approach in a situation are beneficial for handling difficult circumstances.

What has begun to happen in the medical world is an attempt to understand the physiology of how any factors of belief—or spirituality—works. Science has long understood that an emotion such as fear causes certain physiological responses. When confronted with a frightening situation, our hearts race, our palms sweat, and our adrenaline output increases. This reaction may vary, depending on the person's inner ability to approach fear. And this, in turn, is determined in part by a person's DNA, his or her history, whether there has been any training in how to approach fear—for example, the teaching of military, self-defense, and breathing techniques. A person's ability to approach fear is also a product of the spirituality he or she practices.

How we behave—our being—is a product of our belief system. And our belief system is our spirituality, our way of making meaning in the world. A system of belief can be defined as an external entity. Some would even say that there are concepts we learn and take on as a way of believing about or viewing the world. But even how we determine our thoughts is influenced by what we believe to be true and the ways we value the world around us. The expression "spirituality is an inside job" is used to describe our ability to alter our beliefs, attitudes, and ways of making meaning. This is true, regardless of the process a person chooses to nurture and create a spiritual life, whether it is the use of religion, nature, meditation, art, or any of myriad other choices. It begins on the inside.

Spiritual Practices in Patient Care

The role of pastoral care is to determine a person's spiritual beliefs and practices and how they affect his or her ability to cope with illness. Spiritual assessment systems seek to differentiate themselves from other systems by focusing at least primarily on spiritual concerns, as opposed to psychological or social concerns.

Spiritual Assessment

Pruyser (1976) was the first to propose distinctive spiritual care categories to highlight the difference between spiritual and psychological care. Fitchett (1993) proposed a system for pastoral caregivers that allows for a more holistic assessment.

These early systems were comprehensive and covered a full spectrum of spiritual issues, including meaning, hope, relationship to God, ritual, and community. However, their very comprehensiveness makes them unsuitable for acute care settings. More recently, Fitchett (1999) has proposed a distinction between spiritual screening and spiritual assessment. The screening component of this system includes several easily administered questions that can be incorporated into a more global admissions assessment, conducted by a nurse or other member of the health care team. The screening is meant to identify those who could benefit from further assessment and spiritual intervention by pastoral caregivers.

Several paper-and-pencil instruments, such as those described by Kass and others (1991) and Holland and her colleagues (1998), have mainly been used for research purposes but also have been employed to good effect as screening tools in certain settings because they are well correlated with other measures of well-being. In a further step, Holland (1997) and Handzo (1998) have proposed a system that allows a nurse, social worker, or other member of the health care team to quickly screen for psychological, social, and spiritual distress and then refer the patient to the appropriate caregiver for follow-up, based on a preset algorithm. This system also includes a set of spiritual diagnoses, with treatment plans for each. In the fully integrated spiritual care system, the current standard of care includes initial screening on each inpatient admission and periodically in the outpatient setting for spiritual distress and religious needs, with clear guidelines for referral to the appropriate religious or spiritual resources.

At Griffin Hospital in Derby, Connecticut, several approaches to spiritual assessment have been used. Beginning with the admitting process, patients are asked if there is a specific religious community to which they belong, and if so, would they like to have their names listed for that community in order to receive pastoral or spiritual care visits. If they do, then, each morning, a volunteer calls the local religious communities to inform them that one of their members is in the hospital.

Members of the pastoral care department follow up with initial visits to make a spiritual assessment and provide care that is appropriate to the patient's needs. One of the ways Griffin Hospital's pastoral care department has sought to provide a continuum of spiritual care is to link with the parish nurse program, as well as with monthly meetings of the local clergy. If a patient to be discharged has ongoing needs for spiritual care and support, a parish nurse or member of the clergy is contacted for follow-up.

In addition, a mobile health resource van has begun taking a chaplain out into the community, to places where health screenings and health education are provided. A spiritual assessment form has been developed, which is offered along with the cholesterol screening and blood pressure check. Many people served by the mobile health resource van are in need of bereavement counseling, support, and care. These needs can be determined by the chaplain and the spiritual assessment.

Spiritual Interventions

On one level, the interventions used in spiritual care have not changed in hundreds of years. Counseling with a religious professional, studying sacred text, communicating with that which transcends us through prayer or meditation, and using ritual practices, such as worship, have always been with us. What has changed significantly is the way these interventions are applied, especially by pastoral caregivers.

When spiritual care was delivered only by the clergy to members of their own faith group, it was widely assumed that the clergy person would know what the patient needed and would be able to prescribe what he or she should do to alleviate spiritual distress. As modern spiritual care evolved in the twentieth century, it became clear that the appropriate intervention needed to emerge from the patient. The task of spiritual care therefore became to help patients identify and maximize their own spiritual resources rather than bring them into line with what was considered proper by their faith group (Van de Creek and Burton, 2001). This change parallels the movement in medicine to make patients much more active participants in their own care.

Spiritual Counseling

This new approach is nowhere more evident than in the process of the spiritual counseling of those who are in distress. Rather than telling people what they "should" believe, the counselor first assesses in detail what the patient believes about the issues at hand. In the health care setting, these issues usually have to do with the meaning the person wishes to ascribe to his or her suffering, ability to be hopeful, the object(s) of that hope, and how the current situation affects his or her relationship with a higher power.

Finding meaning in events—especially suffering—seems to be a central element in good coping (Park and Folkman, 1997). Religious or spiritual meanings are common choices (Spilka, Shaver, and Kirkpatrick, 1985). In modern spiritual counseling, the goal is to help the sufferer find a meaning that promotes positive coping rather than imposing a meaning that conforms to the generally accepted belief system of the person's faith tradition. Attention needs to be paid not only to the content of the belief but also to its affective component and function for the individual. Individuals who believe that God has caused their illness may be in great distress because the illness means to them that God is punishing them, or they may be comforted because they take the illness as a sign that God is in control. Many Muslims believe that when Allah sends suffering, it is an opportunity to atone for some of their sins and therefore have a better chance of entering heaven. Those providing spiritual counseling need to take care not to impose their own meaning on the patient's beliefs but to attend closely to how a particular belief functions for a particular person.

Often, just as in psychological counseling, the assessment phase itself will lead patients to an understanding about their spiritual concerns. Many patients know what they believe but are concerned because they perceive these beliefs to be divergent from the norm for their faith tradition and therefore "wrong." Affirmation from the counselor that these beliefs are acceptable may be all the person needs to enlist these beliefs in the coping process.

Prayer, Meditation, Visualization

This group of interventions most clearly illustrates the overlap among the traditional practice of pastoral care, modern spiritual care, and treatment techniques normally classed as "psychological." As the concept of what constitutes prayer has moved from prescripted formulations, often said only during a service of worship, to any communication between a person and what he or she conceives to be a higher power, the definitions of prayer and meditation have clearly converged. Whereas prayer is generally conceived of as a dialogue in which the person both speaks and listens, meditation puts the practitioner more clearly into a listening or receiving mode. However, there may be little distinction between praying the rosary, in which the same words are repeated over and over, and the practice of using a mantra in meditation. Benson (1985) points out that religious language functions as an effective focus for meditation if the words have meaning for the person involved.

Today, many spiritual caregivers use meditation and visualization focused on religious or spiritual words and images, among their various treatment options. Work is currently underway to test the use of Psalms as foci for mediation, to improve coping for both religious and nonreligious cancer patients, based on the work of Payne, Lundberg, Brennan, and Holland (1997) and Kabatt-Zinn, Lippworth, and Burney (1985). The spiritual caregiver can assist patients in finding appropriate words or images to use in meditation or visualization as well as in expanding the patient's concept of prayer to make it more useful in coping. Many patients find it more acceptable to use these coping strategies if they are called religious rather than psychological.

Ritual

Just as the definition of prayer has been broadened to encompass a wider range of behaviors, ritual has been redefined to make it useful for a wider range of patients. Driver (1991), among others, has recognized the importance of ritual outside of purely religious contexts. Probably because the mechanism of action is not clearly understood, the power of ritual has been vastly underestimated, especially in coping with suffering and loss. However, many people turn to ritual as a way of coping.

Ritual in spiritual care falls into two categories. The first encompasses set rituals from the person's faith tradition. Patients often return to the rituals of their childhood religion, even when they have otherwise disavowed it. The mother of a teenaged boy who was newly diagnosed with cancer had converted years earlier from Roman Catholicism to Protestantism because the rituals had no meaning for her. Yet she asked to have a Catholic priest bless her son with holy water. A Jewish patient who had practiced his faith as a child, but had not done so for most of his life, began to cry when a traditional prayer for healing was said in Hebrew. A Muslim patient was upset because he was unable to perform the physical movements that accompany his daily prayer. Many patients who have regularly attended worship in their faith tradition are upset when unable to do so.

Caregivers need to assess what rituals might be important to patients in maintaining the feeling of normalcy in their lives or in giving them a sense of control over their situation. When patients are unable to perform normal rituals because of their physical state or hospital regulation, a chaplain may be helpful in creating a comparable ritual. In the case of the Muslim patient, the Imam explained to him that imaging the movements in his mind while praying was equivalent in the eyes of Allah to actually doing them. As patients in health care institutions become sicker and thus less able to attend worship services of their faith, services on individual nursing units or over in-house television become increasingly important.

It is often helpful to be able to improvise rituals to deal with specific circumstances. In the recovery of bodies from the World Trade Center, complex rituals evolved for the handling of each body, assuring all involved that the deceased was being treated with respect. Many neonatal units have developed ritualized procedures to help parents begin to grieve their loss. Van der Hart (1988) has written extensively about devising particular rituals, especially for coping with specific losses.

Interdisciplinary Contributions

The pastoral caregiver in the current health care environment represents the spiritual dimension of care not only for patients and families but also for the entire health care team and the institution itself. Chaplains do not provide all the spiritual care any more than the psychologist provides all the emotional care, but they do provide an expert resource for the patient, the patient's loved ones, and the staff in using spiritual resources to cope with loss and suffering. After the World Trade Center attack, chaplains in many health care institutions offered worship services and other rituals for the staff. Many of these were well attended, even in institutions with no tradition of this practice.

Pastoral caregivers are also important participants on hospital ethics committees and institutional review boards. Besides representing religious and cultural beliefs and values, chaplains represent a nonmedical voice that helps others see issues from a lay person's point of view.

Spiritual Care at Griffin Hospital: A Case Study

In addition to the interventions previously discussed, at Griffin Hospital, the pastoral care department has initiated the redesign of the Interfaith Chapel, which includes a waterfall and the playing of quiet music. A prayer book is kept open so that people can write their prayers and thoughts into it. There are resources for a variety of faith traditions within the chapel while maintaining a neutral and sacred space for anyone to stop by for a quiet moment of meditation or prayer.

At Griffin Hospital, spirituality is integrated into the entire hospital. One of the ways this is accomplished is through attention to the environment. The soothing effect of the surroundings enhances spiritual comfort. For most people, being able to hear music, provided through the arts and entertainment program, is a welcome relief and release. Hearing a piano, violin, or guitar playing quietly in the background can heighten a person's sense of peace and calm.

The volunteer baking program in each kitchen on the medical units provides the comforting smell of cookies, bread, and muffins. Most patients and visitors comment that Griffin, with the music playing and the nursing units open with flowers on the tables and fish tanks in the waiting areas, does not seem like a hospital. All of these environmental touches create an atmosphere of serenity and peace, which, in turn, gives patients and family members a sense of comfort and calm. Seeking a calming and serene sense of self is not just a physical need; it also serves to create an atmosphere that permeates the inner spiritual self. The environment itself becomes a symbol of mind, body, and spirit.

Planetree Spirituality

All Planetree affiliates start with an understanding that patient care encompasses mind, body, and spirit. Each affiliate addresses spiritual care differently. Most have an interfaith chapel, which provides a sacred and quiet space for patients, families, and employees. To acknowledge the important role of caregivers, many Planetree affiliates have established a ritual for the Blessing of Hands, which is provided by going throughout the hospital to include all the staff. For some affiliates, this is part of the Planetree retreat.

The chaplain at Columbia Memorial Hospital has developed a series of classes for interested staff members, to help them become more aware of the impact that spirituality has on health and well-being. The three one-hour sessions include experiential exercises, discussions regarding the difference between spirituality and religion, and an overview of world religions. The purpose of the classes is to give staff members greater insight into their own spirituality so that they can be more attentive to the spiritual needs of the patients.

Banner Health System, which includes health care facilities in Arizona and Colorado, has developed a variety of creative means for addressing spiritual care. A portable labyrinth, used for meditation, can be taken to various sites. In another setting within Banner, the Clinical Pastoral Education program has obtained grant monies to create a pastoral and spiritual training program for bilingual Hispanic chaplains. With this special initiative, the program is better able to meet the spiritual needs of the third of its patients who are Spanish-speaking.

In another Banner facility, the chaplain (who is of the Sikh tradition) created a beautiful banner with the words "Let us pray" in the twenty different languages spoken by the staff members. People were invited to a ritual where they were asked to write "Let us pray" in their native language. The banner was hung in the chapel and a photograph of it was made into a bookmark to be given to all patients.

Because spirituality and ritual are an integral part of healing in the Navajo tradition, Page Hospital in Page, Arizona, is building a ceremonial hogan on hospital grounds. The hogan will enable Navajo practitioners to use ceremonial smoke, herbs, and fire to provide a healing center for the 68 percent of patients at Page who are Native American. Walking around the circular hogan, symbolic for traveling life's journey, is seen as helping to restore health and harmony.

End-of-life care brings additional spiritual needs. The hospice at Wellmont Bristol Regional Medical Center in Bristol, Tennessee, has linked with local churches to provide support for hospice families and caregivers. Each month, a different church stocks the family kitchen with snack foods and staples and provides care packages for all patients in the hospice program—both inpatients and outpatients. Prayer cards are provided for patients as well as for the hospice staff, often with the name of the church member who is praying for them.

At Wellmont Holston Valley Medical Center in Kingsport, Tennessee, patients who choose to be admitted to an "intensive prayer unit" can include prayer in their plan of care.

A bereavement program was established by Northside Hospital in Atlanta, Georgia, to provide spiritual care after the death of an employee or an employee's close family member. A personal letter of condolence from the CEO is sent to the employee or family. A bereavement package is provided with information about benefits, insurance, and Northside's employee assistance program, which is available to employees' families as well. Information is included to help with the grieving process. To express their respect for members of the Northside "family," staff members, managers, and administrators are encouraged to attend the funerals. At the one-year anniversary of a death, a beautifully wrapped votive candle, with a prayer attached, is given to the employee or family.

Catskill Regional Medical Center in Harris, New York, implemented a "White Rose" program to honor patients who have died. After a death, a white silk rose is placed on the patient's pillow, privacy curtain, or door out of respect for the patient and as a means of communicating to other caregivers that a death has occurred. The rose is then given to the family as a keepsake.

Kane Community Hospital provides spiritual care twenty-four hours a day, seven days a week, through its volunteer chaplain service. Local pastors rotate as the on-call chaplain. Framed signs in the emergency department and other waiting areas list the phone number and encourage patients, family members, and staff members to call any time they would like to speak with a chaplain. Chaplains also provide Sunday and holiday services for those who may be unable to attend regular services.

Patient care is, by its very nature, spiritual. Although Planetree hospitals differ in how they address the spiritual needs of patients, families, and staff members, being sensitive to traditions and cultures, as well as to religious and spiritual practices, is a primary goal. The purpose of spiritual care is to honor the whole person and all that a person's life reflects.

References

Benson, H. *Beyond the Relaxation Response*. New York: Berkeley Books, 1985.

Driver, T. *The Magic of Ritual: Our Need for Liberating Rites That Transform Our Lives and Communities*. New York: HarperCollins, 1991.

Fitchett, G. *Assessing Spiritual Needs: A Guide for Caregivers*. Minneapolis: Augsburg Fortress Press, 1993.

Fitchett, G. "Screening for Spiritual Risk." *Chaplaincy Today*, 1999, 15(1), 2–12.

Handzo, G. "An Integrated System for the Assessment and Treatment of Psychological, Social, and Spiritual Distress." *Chaplaincy Today*, 1998, 14(2), 30–37.

Holland, J. C. "Preliminary Guidelines for the Treatment of Distress." *Oncology*, 1997, 11(11A), 109–114.

Holland, J. C., and others. "A Brief Spiritual Beliefs Inventory for Use in Quality of Life Research in Life-Threatening Illness." *Psycho-Oncology*, 1998, 7(1), 460–469.

Kabatt-Zinn, J., Lippworth, L., and Burney, R. "The Clinical Uses of Mindfulness Meditation for the Self-Regulation of Chronic Pain." *Journal of Behavioral Medicine*, 1985, 8, 163–190.

Kass, J., and others. "Health Outcomes and a New Index of Spiritual Experience." *Journal for the Scientific Study of Religion*, 1991, 30(2), 203–211.

Mueller, P., and Plevak, D. "Religious Involvement, Spirituality, and Medicine: Complications for Clinical Practice." *Mayo Clinical Procedures*, 2001, 76, 1.

Park, C., and Folkman, S. "Meaning in the Context of Stress and Coping." *Review of General Psychology*, 1997, 1(2), 115–144.

Payne, D., Lundberg, J., Brennan, M., and Holland, J. "A Psychosocial Intervention for Patients with Soft Tissue Sarcoma." *Psycho-Oncology*, 1997, 6, 65–71.

Pruyser, P. *The Minister as Diagnostician*. Philadelphia: Westminster Press, 1976.

Siegel, B. "Spirituality in Medicine." Lecture, Ann Arbor, Mich., 1984.

Spilka, B., Shaver, P., and Kirkpatrick, L. "A General Attribution Theory of the Psychology of Religion." *Journal of the Scientific Study of Religion*, 1985, 24(1), 1–118.

Van de Creek, L., and Burton, L. "Professional Chaplaincy: Its Role and Importance in Healthcare." *Journal of Pastoral Care*, 2001, 55(1), 81–97.

Van der Hart, O. (ed.). *The Therapeutic Use of Leave-Taking Rituals*. New York: Irvington, 1988.

6

Human Touch

The Essentials of Communicating Caring Through Massage

Michele Spatz with Dianne Storby

Massage has played an integral part in the Planetree model of patient-centered care over the past twenty years. One of the first hospital-based massage and massage training programs began at a Planetree-model hospital in California. As the American public has rediscovered the health benefits of massage, Planetree hospitals have found innovative ways to incorporate it as a staple in delivering good patient care.

Massage is a powerful way to communicate caring, and it was once an essential element of good nursing care. Unfortunately, it has been largely forgotten in the high-pressured world of modern medicine, where regulation, documentation, and staff shortages leave too little time for patient contact. The experience of illness is often frightening, and the treatment of illness, particularly in the hospital, is even more so. Massage offers a profound means of balancing a hospital's intimidating environment with the gentleness of human touch. Massage for nurses, doctors, and other hospital staff members is equally important in caring for those who care for others.

History of Massage Therapy

Massage used therapeutically is as old as antiquity. There are historic records of massage being incorporated into Eastern medicine as early as 2700 B.C. Some believe that its origins are in intuitive human contact, much as mammals in nature instinctively touch and stroke each other (Holey and Cook, 1997). Even Hippocrates, the father of modern Western medicine, used massage to treat his patients, and he advised, "The physician must be acquainted with many things and assuredly with rubbing . . . for rubbing can bind a joint that is too loose or loosen a joint that is too hard" (Fritz, 1995, p. 5).

Massage was introduced in the United States in the 1850s by two physician brothers, George and Charles Taylor, who studied it in Sweden. It wasn't long before the first massage therapy clinics opened in the United States, shortly following the Civil War. Massage was historically considered a medical tool, but by the early 1900s medicine had become a more formalized science. Physicians became time-pressed as a result of new medical technologies, methods, and procedures used to treat their patients, and so they delegated responsibility for massage to nurses or assistants. As the demands on nurses grew, massage disappeared entirely from the medical setting by the mid-1900s and was then practiced outside it. Oddly, it evolved from accepted medical practice into an "alternative therapy" (Holey and Cook, 1997). Fortunately, the pendulum is swinging back to incorporate massage as a healing modality into the hospital and patient care setting. There is a renaissance in recognizing the importance of touch to healing. We know through clinical research that massage offers documented health benefits. It has reestablished itself as an important health care tool, and it speaks profoundly to a most basic human need—to be touched and comforted. In the vulnerable world of the hospital, touch connects patients to their innermost selves, has therapeutic value, and builds a meaningful bond between caregiver and patient.

Training Requirements

Training requirements for massage therapists vary by state and may be determined by state statutes or governed by a state regulatory agency. Currently, thirty states and the District of Columbia regulate massage. The American Massage Therapy Association requires its members to complete a minimum training of 500 hours of classroom instruction from a school that is accredited by the Commission on Massage Therapy Accreditation. The commission itself requires that accredited massage therapy schools provide at least 120 hours of coursework in anatomy, physiology, and pathology and a minimum of 100 hours of supervised hands-on practice, in addition to a student's fieldwork or clinic work. Accredited schools must include a curriculum that covers the history, theory, technique, and practice of massage therapy as well as addressing contraindications, the benefits of massage, standard precautions, body mechanics, the legalities of massage, and professional standards regarding draping and modesty.

Once training is complete, massage therapists may be certified by the National Certification Board for Therapeutic Massage and Bodywork after successfully passing its National Certification Examination. Recertification through this voluntary program is required every four years and involves submitting documentation of the completion of two hundred or more work hours, coupled with fifty hours of continuing education. Successfully completing the current National Certification Examination may substitute for the continuing education requirement toward recertification.

Literature on the Therapeutic Value of Massage in the Hospital Setting

There is much research to support the therapeutic value of massage for a multitude of ailments—from helping to cope with chronic obstructive pulmonary disease (COPD) to restoring normal cardiac rhythm to relieve pain. Richards, Gibson, and Overton-McCoy (2000) examined the effect of massage on hospital patients in acute and critical care settings. Their review shows a decrease in anxiety, an increase in physical relaxation, and a reduction in pain among patients receiving massage. A study by Smith, Stallings, Mariner, and Burrall (1999) found that hospitalized patients who received one to four massages during the course of their hospital stay reported an increase in relaxation, a greater sense of well-being, and positive mood changes. Billhult and Dahlberg (2001) report in their small study on the use of massage on hospitalized female cancer patients that massage offered the patients "a meaningful relief from suffering."

Massage is also an integral part of caring for the caregiver. Katz, Wowk, Culp, and Wakeling (1999) found in their pilot study of registered nurses who received fifteen-minute massages during the workday that pain intensity and tension levels were significantly lowered after the massage. Further results showed improved levels of relaxation and positive mood state after the massage. In the health care setting, massage is a beneficial tool for reducing workplace stress and taking good care of caregivers.

Model Massage Therapy Programs: Mid-Columbia Medical Center

In November 1996, Mid-Columbia Medical Center (MCMC), a Planetree hospital in The Dalles, Oregon, opened its Center for Mind and Body, offering a holistic, patient-centered approach to improving the quality of life for individuals with chronic illnesses. Massage has been offered at MCMC since 1992, yet its delivery became more fully integrated into patient care environments with the advent of the Center for Mind and Body. Several licensed massage therapists were hired as part-time hospital employees at this time, offering massage to patients and health care workers throughout the hospital in a variety of innovative ways.

Same-Day Surgery

At MCMC, every patient scheduled for surgery is offered a massage. After arrival in the department, patients are assigned a room in which to change their clothing, have their vital signs checked, and complete any necessary paperwork before their operation or procedure. During the waiting period before transport, time often fraught with anxiety, massage therapists "round" from room to room and offer a brief massage. Patients who agree to the service sit in comfortable recliners while the therapist delivers a ten-minute head and neck, arms, hands, and shoulder massage. For patient comfort and ease of delivery, the massage is given through the patient's gown. This simple act of prescribed touch communicates to patients on a profound level that they are not alone—there are others who care and are along with them on their healing journey. Many patients express relief and have shared how beneficial having a massage prior to surgery was for them. Most often, patients will comment that it helped them relax and reduced their anxiety. It is a beautiful gift to the patients, helping them release muscle tension and connecting them to the art and comfort of being cared for.

"Beth" was diagnosed with bilateral breast cancer in June 2001. She was offered massage by her surgeon as part of a package of services available to her as a new cancer patient at MCMC. Prior to her surgery, she felt "very nervous, anxious, worried about what they were going to find there. It was very stressful."

She was offered a presurgery massage, which she describes as "so relaxing that I realized I was very ready to fight this disease and go into surgery with a good attitude." Her advice is that "every patient should at least try it."

Sharon, a licensed massage therapist at MCMC, offers this perspective on presurgery massages: "Most of the patients are somewhat nervous. I think of it as varying degrees of nervousness. The massage for them seems to be really soothing—something that soothes them and gets their mind off of their impending surgery. It has a calming effect. Because massage is a nurturing therapy, it helps establish trust by connecting patients and their caregivers. I think the patients realize on a deep level, 'Okay, this is a hospital person and these people are going to take care of me. The surgery is going to be okay because the people are going to be taking care of me in there, too.'"

Acute Care Units

Hospitalized patients are admitted for a variety of medical problems on the acute care in-patient floor, many of whom respond positively to massage therapy. The American Massage Therapy Association lists arthritis, asthma, carpal tunnel syndrome, chronic and acute pain, circulatory problems, gastrointestinal disorders, headache, immune function disorders, insomnia, myofascial pain, reduced range of motion, strained muscles and ligaments, stress, and temporo-mandibular joint syndrome as conditions shown to respond to massage therapy (see the American Massage Therapy Association Web site: http://amtamassage.org/about/physicians.htm). Many of the health benefits of massage and its application to science and medicine are being studied and archived by the Touch Research Institute (TRI) at the University of Miami's School of Medicine (http://www.miami.edu/touch-research). Among the discoveries is the effectiveness of massage in reducing pain and stress, boosting the immune system, and improving weight gain in premature babies, leading to their earlier discharge. In addition to its powerful healing properties, massage offers a comfort measure to patients who are coping with a new and often frightening environment.

At MCMC, patients on the acute care floor are offered massage through a variety of mechanisms. As nurses perform their initial assessment of a new patient, they enter the demographics, physical signs, symptoms, and patient medical history into a handheld computer. The patient assessment software on the nurse's handheld computer also prompts them to offer the patient a massage. If the patient responds positively, the nurse enters this into the handheld computer. The massage therapist is notified to visit the patient by a request, which is automatically generated by the handheld computer and routed to the massage therapist. Physicians also order massages for their patients because they see massage as an integral part of care and caring. However, a physician's order is not required for massage therapy to be administered. Patients themselves may self-refer and request a massage. And, of course, massage therapists on duty will visit acute care patients and offer their services.

Licensed massage therapist Sharon states, "It's been surprising to me over and over again to see people who are really uncomfortable and either in pain or just not feeling well in some way; it's been a surprise to me that they *want* the massage. Usually, you think they just don't want to be touched, but that's simply not so. That nurturing and feel-good touch, 99 percent of the time, does help them feel better."

Sharon shares a story about massage making a difference in a patient's hospital experience. "An older woman with COPD was literally down on the floor on her knees, leaning on her hospital bed when I walked into her room. She was absolutely miserable. She was having trouble breathing and the reason she was down on the floor was because her back hurt so badly, she just couldn't be in the bed any longer. She had never had a massage before, so I started working on her just as she was—kneeling on the floor, leaning against the bed. She couldn't believe how good it felt. After a while, she let me help her back into her bed. I finished the massage with her in the bed. I really don't have words to describe her transformation. She was so thankful."

Celilo Center for Cancer Care

MCMC's Celilo Center offers the best of cancer treatment by using state-of-the-art science and technology to treat the physical symptoms of cancer and incorporating time-tested complementary therapies, such as massage, to reduce stress and bolster the immune system function. It is an integrated mind, spirit, and whole-body approach, and patients love it.

Judi, an oncology nurse who is also a licensed massage therapist (LMT), gives head, neck, feet, hands, and shoulder massages to chemotherapy patients while they are receiving their infusions. This service is presently provided one day per week and is extended to family members accompanying loved ones to treatment, providing often-needed comfort to worn-out caregivers. Lymphatic drainage massage is being added to the LMT's repertoire for treatment of patients with lymphedema, as recent studies indicate that it is an effective treatment modality (Cohen, Payne, and Tunkel, 2001; Erickson and others, 2001).

Celilo nurses talk about how helpful the massage therapist is at putting patients at ease when they are in distress. Because massage offers one-on-one attention and a distraction, Judi is the first caregiver they employ for a difficult patient. Often, chemotherapy patients will confide in Judi because she is perceived as having time to listen. According to Lyn, registered nurse and care manager for Celilo Center, "Judi makes more of a difference with the patients than anyone else on the unit. She is able to relax them and spend time with them, and they trust her. Patients will tell Judi about their side effects that they won't share with the medical or nursing staff. She is a calming influence and the doctors and nurses are perceived as more fearsome. Judi will ask patients, 'What's the scoop?' and they tell her." Judi is able to share a patient's clinically relevant information with the medical staff in order to improve patient comfort and care. Chemotherapy nurses report that patients want to schedule their chemotherapy *only* on "Judi day."

Wendy, a non-Hodgkins lymphoma patient, says she came to her first chemotherapy appointment "feeling apprehensive. I was worried about side effects." She was offered a massage during her first chemotherapy visit and she requested a foot massage, which she found "very relaxing." During a difficult time in her treatment, she wasn't sleeping well, so she decided to use massage therapy at home. Her son massaged her feet at night and it relaxed her to the point of sleep.

Beth, undergoing chemotherapy for her breast cancer, states, "There is so much goodwill and great vibes at Celilo. Massage is just one more thing to help you relax. Many people are afraid of needles and you know you are not going to be feeling well. Massage helps the time go faster and it relieves a lot of stress." When asked, Beth is not sure where her outlet of stress would have gone if massage therapy had not been available. She believes she would not have healed as quickly.

Patients are not the only ones to benefit from massage therapy at Celilo. Oncology is demanding work, so Judi also offers brief head, neck, and shoulder massages to the Celilo staff. "All she has to do is touch me and I'm able to let go. She transports us and takes us away from here," says Lyn. "It's intoxicating."

Radiation therapy patients are also offered head, neck, hands, and shoulder massages. They may choose to receive their massage either before or after their radiation treatment. Again, family members are also extended an invitation for a massage. Many patients and their family members express regret at the end of their active treatment phase because they will miss their massage. In order for patients to continue to receive its benefits, they may follow up and schedule a private massage with any of the hospital staff therapists through the Center for Mind and Body. Massages are offered at cost only and are given in secluded, peaceful massage rooms at Celilo Center.

Infant Massage

Recently, a certified infant massage therapist was added to the MCMC staff. She offers parents an opportunity to learn infant massage through the hospital's postpartum clinic. Infant massage has been shown to increase weight gain among premature infants, result in less crying among full-term infants, and increase parent-infant bonding (Zlotnick, 2000). Other avenues to share infant massage with parents are being developed, including training hospital employees whose children attend the facility's day care center and offering community classes.

Employee Massage

Those who care for others often carry a great responsibility. Practicing in today's health care setting is fraught with paperwork, staff shortages, and myriad rules and regulations. At MCMC, massage is offered to employees as an effective stress reduction tool. While massage therapists are working on a patient care unit, they offer quick five- to ten-minute massages to the staff. For willing employees, a head, neck, shoulder, and arm massage is given at the workstation, through work clothes. A department director may also call and request that massage therapy services be delivered to departmental employees. This service is particularly valuable on high-stress days or after emotionally draining events. Managers may also offer employees simple massages during departmental retreats as a way to give to and thank their health care workers. During retreats, massage therapists travel the room and offer short neck and shoulder massages to participants. For special events or for reward and recognition, massage gift certificates are also given to employees.

Overcoming Obstacles

As wonderful as massage therapy is in the hospital setting, there are challenges to its successful integration. Some physician resistance early on is not uncommon. Generally this has to do with the confusion of trained, licensed massage therapists with masseuses working in "massage parlors." As physicians themselves experience the relaxing effects of massage therapy and witness the dramatic shift in their patients' comfort level and disposition, resistance evaporates.

Perhaps the most significant obstacle is the fact that massage therapy is not yet reimbursable by most insurance companies. The question becomes How do you pay for this service? Knowing that there was not going to be reimbursement for services but believing it was the right thing to offer patients, MCMC planned its massage therapy program as a noncost recovery service. Every hospital has some degree of flexibility in designating "overhead" or "loss leader" services that may make indirect contributions to the bottom line. The total annual budget for the massage therapy program at MCMC is approximately $125,000. Massage therapy can be viewed as a valued part of a comprehensive program to meet each patient's medical, psychological, and spiritual needs during his or her hospital stay. The investment in providing such a service pays great dividends in the form of higher patient satisfaction, patient share, and market share.

Massage therapy in the hospital setting is such a recent phenomenon that recruitment can be a challenge. It may be difficult to find massage therapists who have received adequate training to work with patients—especially oncology patients. In addition, it takes a special person to be comfortable in the hospital environment. When asked why she chose massage therapy, after having been a certified nurse's assistant for many years, Sharon, now a licensed massage therapist, says, "I wanted to combine nurturing with being in the hospital setting. The patients are so appreciative. It's just a feel-good kind of job." Sharon describes the main difference between hospital massage work and that in non-hospital settings as "my own body mechanics. I work around machines, tubes, and equipment as well as the positions the patients are able to be in."

Healing Environments

Healing human touch can be offered in all health care environments—from the chemotherapy infusion center, to inpatient rooms, to staff areas. In planning an environment most conductive to massage therapy, some of the most important elements to consider are availability of a quiet place, subdued lighting, and soft music.

However, a more open approach to massage in some clinical settings can have unanticipated benefits. For example, one day in the Celilo Center chemotherapy room, Judi offered a massage to Arnold, a patient with metastatic bladder cancer. He was bald, so Judi asked if he wanted her to massage his head. He agreed and Judi put her massage lotion on his head and began to gently massage him. Seeing him visibly relax, Tammy, a breast cancer patient who had lost her hair and was very shy about her baldness, whipped off her hat and asked for her bald head to be massaged next. It was an important moment for Tammy to reveal herself to the others, in the most light-hearted of ways, by simply throwing off her cap and announcing, "Next!" Like dominoes, other patients in the room followed suit.

Typically, hospitals are not places where people want to spend much time, and cancer centers are particularly dreaded places. Yet many patients report that their family members vie to accompany them to their Celilo appointments because they know that they will be treated to a simple massage. The use of therapeutic massage is a critical element that transforms the healing environment. "Massage is valuable in the hospital from the feedback I get from patients," states Sharon, MCMC licensed massage therapist. "They mention how wonderful it was and how other hospitals they have been to should be doing the same thing and how they are telling other people. The patients are spreading the word."

Through their vision and commitment to patient-centered care, many Planetree hospitals have successfully integrated the ancient art of massage therapy into the delivery of modern Western medical care. Although not often a revenue-generating service, the sense of connection massage therapy offers between caregiver and patient, coupled with its healing influence, makes it priceless.

References

Billhult, A., and Dahlberg, K. "A Meaningful Relief from Suffering: Experiences of Massage in Cancer Care." *Cancer Nursing*, 2001, *24*(3), 180–184.

Cohen, S. R., Payne, D. K., and Tunkel, R. S. "Lymphedema: Strategies for Management." *Cancer*, 2001, *92* (supp. 4), 980–987.

Erickson, V. S., and others. "Arm Edema in Breast Cancer Patients." *Journal of the National Cancer Institute*, 2001, *93*(2), 96–111.

Fritz, S. *Mosby's Fundamentals of Therapeutic Massage*. St. Louis, Mo.: Mosby-Year Book, 1995.

Holey, E., and Cook, E. *Therapeutic Massage*. Philadelphia, Pa.: Saunders, 1997.

Katz, J., Wowk, A., Culp, D., and Wakeling, H. "Pain and Tension Are Reduced Among Hospital Nurses After On-Site Massage Treatments: A Pilot Study." *Journal of Perianesthesia Nursing*, 1999, *14*(3), 128–133.

Richards, K. C., Gibson, R., and Overton-McCoy, A. L. "Effects of Massage in Acute and Critical Care." *AACN Clinical Issues*, 2000, *11*(1), 77–96.

Smith, M. C., Stallings, M. A., Mariner, S., and Burrall, M. "Benefits of Massage Therapy for Hospitalized Patients: A Descriptive and Qualitative Evaluation." *Alternative Therapies in Health and Medicine*, 1999, *5*(4), 64–71.

Zlotnick, M. "Infant Massage: Building Relationships Through Touch." *International Journal of Childbirth Education*, 2000, *15*(1), 36–38.

7

Healing Arts
Nutrition for the Soul

Roger Ulrich and Laura Gilpin

L ong before science was synonymous with medicine, the arts and healing were closely and intricately intertwined. In the centuries before Hippocrates, the healing temples of ancient Greece surrounded patients with music, poetry, storytelling, painting, sculpture, gardens, and fountains. An environment rich with art was seen as therapeutic, providing a means to alleviate physical discomfort, emotional distress, and spiritual crisis. In the absence of science, the arts were vital in restoring the will to live and enhancing the healing process.

With the advent of science, the therapeutic uses of the arts diminished in importance but were still perceived intuitively to enhance healing. Florence Nightingale, in her classic book *Notes on Nursing* ([1860] 1969), describes the patient's need for beauty, even to look out a window or gaze at a vase of flowers: "People say the effect is only on the mind. It is no such thing. The effect is on the body, too. Little as we know about the way in which we are affected by form, by colour, and light, we do know this, that they have an actual physical effect. Variety of form and brilliancy of colour in the objects presented to patients are actual means of recovery" (p. 59.)

For many patients, illness and hospitalization can be a time of pain, fear, anxiety, and loneliness. Despite the incredible advances in the science of medicine, or perhaps because of them, hospitals, with their life-saving equipment, procedures, and technologies, have become sterile, intimidating institutions.

But science does not preclude the arts. The Planetree model was founded on the belief that science is best delivered in an environment most conducive to healing. The first Planetree unit provided patients with a wide variety of arts, including music, painting, storytelling, movies, clowns, juggling, and volunteers to engage the patients in creative expression.

Ironically, the arts have come full circle. The science that once overshadowed the arts is now verifying their importance. Western medicine is now finding evidence for what was felt intuitively centuries ago: that the arts can play a vital role in speeding recovery.

At first inspection, health care professionals may view the involvement of art and music as peripheral, but there now exists scientific research linking art in health care facilities to improved medical outcomes. In particular, the effects of viewing art (paintings, prints, photographs) on stress reduction and other medical outcomes has been a growing area of investigation.

For purposes of clarity, one must first define a key term—*medical outcome,* and explain why evidence from research on arts/outcomes relationships should inform art selection for health care facilities. There exist science-grounded theories for understanding why certain categories and styles of art consistently tend to improve medical outcomes, whereas other types of art may sometimes engender negative reactions and accordingly be inappropriate for patients.

What Is a Health Outcome?

An important term relevant to arts/health research is *health outcome,* which refers to the measure of a patient's condition or progress or is an indicator of health care quality (Ulrich, 1999, 2002). There are different types of health or medical outcomes, including

- Clinical indicators that are observable signs and symptoms relating to patients' conditions (examples: length of hospital stay, blood pressure, intake of pain medication)

- Patient-/staff-/family-based outcomes (examples: patient ratings of perceived pain, patient reports of satisfaction with health care services, staff-reported satisfaction with working conditions)

- Economic outcomes (examples: cost of patient care, recruitment or hiring costs due to staff turnover, philanthropy to hospital)

Different combinations of outcomes are used for studying patients with different types of diagnoses. If the objective is to research the effects of artwork on patients recovering from surgery, for example, relevant medical outcomes could include recovery indicators such as reported pain, intake of pain medication, how soon before the patient can move or walk, and length of hospital stay.

Outcome studies have major importance in medicine because they provide the most sound and widely accepted basis for judging whether particular treatments or interventions (art, here) are medically effective and cost-efficient. As health care providers face mounting pressures to control costs yet increase care quality, outcomes research is becoming more influential than ever in affecting decisions and expenditures. The future role and importance of art in health care facilities will without question be strongly affected by the extent to which sound and credible research shows that art can promote improved clinical indicators and enhance patient/consumer satisfaction with providers (Ulrich, 1999).

Outcome studies are also important for helping physicians and medical professionals evaluate whether medical treatments or interventions are *ethical*. The ethics of displaying a given artwork in a museum or workplace is only occasionally an important consideration. Ethics become an overriding consideration, however, when art is displayed to a captive population of vulnerable patients who are stressed, fearful, and in pain. A key dictum that all medical students learn comes from the Hippocratic oath: "First do no harm." The obligation ethically and professionally in the case of art, therefore, is to provide evidence, or at least a chain of plausible reasoning, that the art intervention will cause little or no harm and have positive effects on the great majority of patients (Ulrich, 2002). Adverse reactions to the art should be mild and should occur at acceptably low rates, as virtually any medical intervention may trigger some adverse reactions (Martin, 1999).

Although some artists and designers may assume that nearly any type of visual art or painting is "good" and will beneficially affect patients, it must be kept in mind that artwork varies enormously, and the content and styles of much art are challenging or strongly emotional (Ulrich, 1986). Accordingly, it is reasonable to expect that certain types of art will be positive for patients, whereas other types could be stressful and could worsen outcomes (Ulrich, 1991; Marberry, 1995). The decisive criterion for health care art is whether it improves patient outcomes, not whether it receives praise from art critics and artists or approaches museum standards for quality (Ulrich, 1991, 1999; Marberry, 1995; Martin, 1999; Friedrich, 1999).

Theories: Types of Art That Reduce Stress and Promote Improved Outcomes

Two different theoretical perspectives, *evolutionary congruence* and *emotional congruence*, are helpful in understanding the types of art that have been found effective in improving outcomes.

Evolutionary Theory: Why Nature Art Reduces Stress

The intuitively based belief that viewing nature can be calming, reduce stress, and promote health dates back many centuries and appears across Asian and Western cultures (Ulrich and Parsons, 1992; Ulrich and others, 1991). Writers traditionally attributed this belief to culture and individual and group learning, arguing that societies teach or condition their populations to revere nature and rural scenery but perceive cities and built areas as stressful and negative (Ulrich and Parsons, 1992). Cultural explanations have proven inadequate, however, for explaining the mounting scientific evidence that a diversity of cultures and socioeconomic groups exhibits striking agreement in responding positively to nature views (Ulrich, 1993; Coss, forthcoming). Compared with cultural explanations, evolutionary theory readily accounts for this similarity by proposing that millions of years of evolution have left a genetic mark on modern humans in terms of a predisposition to respond positively to nature settings that fostered well-being and survival (Appleton, 1975; Wilson, 1984; Orians, 1986; Kaplan and Kaplan, 1989; Ulrich, 1983; Coss, forthcoming).

Much of the writings on evolutionary theory have focused on understanding aesthetic preferences for nature, but this theory is also useful in explaining why certain types of nature views and art should have stress-reducing, healthful effects. In this regard, Ulrich (1993; Ulrich and others, 1991) has proposed that the advantages of recovery (restoration from stress) were so critical for the survival of early humans as to favor the selection of individuals with a partly genetic capacity for responding to certain nature settings. This hardwired predisposition would have enhanced survival chances by promoting faster recovery from the fatiguing, unhealthful stress consequences of flight-or-fight behaviors that were essential for dealing successfully with daily threats and demanding situations. From this it follows that as a carryover from evolution, modern humans are predisposed to experience restoration when viewing certain nature content, such as vegetation or water, but not when viewing most built or "modern" materials, such as concrete (Ulrich, 1993, 1999). This evolutionary thinking is consistent with research discussed in a later section showing that certain nature art can effectively produce restoration, even in acutely stressed hospital patients.

Evolutionary theory suggests that nature art will promote restoration across diverse groups of people if it contains the following features and properties: calm or slowly moving water, verdant foliage, flowers, foreground spatial openness, park-like or savannah-like properties (scattered trees, grassy understory), and birds or other unthreatening wildlife (Ulrich, 1993, 1999; Coss, forthcoming).

Furthermore, evolutionary theory proposes that in addition to such nature art, humans are genetically predisposed to pay attention to, and be positively affected by, images of smiling or sympathetic human faces (Darwin, [1872] 1965; Ekman, Friesen, and Ellsworth, 1972). The evolutionary importance of sensitivity to faces and facial expressions of emotion is highlighted by research showing that, for example, newborn human infants are sensitive to faces and even simple face-like sketches (Johnson, Dziurawiec, Ellis, and Morton, 1991; Easterbrook, Kisilevsky, Hains, and Muir, 1999).

Finally, evolutionary theory is useful for identifying features and subject matter that should be *avoided* when selecting art for stressed patients. Speaking generally, an evolutionary perspective holds that humans have a partly innate predisposition to respond negatively (with stress, fear, avoidance behavior) to natural elements and situations that have signaled threats or dangers throughout evolution (Coss, 1968; Ulrich, 1993; Ulrich and others, 1991). These disturbing and often stressful stimuli include snakes and spiders, reptilian-like tessellated scale patterns, nearby large mammals staring directly at the viewer, pointed or piercing forms, shadowy enclosed spaces, and angry or fearful human faces (Öhman, 1986; Coss, 1968, forthcoming; Ulrich, 1993). Findings from several studies of identical twins have left no doubt that genetic factors play a major role in fear responses to certain visual stimuli, such as snakes (for example, Kendler, Karkowski, and Prescott, 1999). This partly genetic underpinning underscores the importance of excluding art containing such phenomena from health care spaces where stress is a problem.

Emotional Congruence Theory: Effects of Patient Emotions on Art Perceptions

In addition to evolutionary theory, another perspective that is quite useful for understanding patient responses to health care art is that of *emotional congruence theory*. Much research in the behavioral sciences has shown that emotions or feelings have important effects on perception and thinking. From this work has emerged emotional congruence theory—the notion that peoples' emotional states bias their perception of environmental stimuli and information in ways that match their feelings (Bower, 1981; Singer and Salovey, 1988; Niedenthal, Setterlund, and Jones, 1994). Other research indicates that emotional states can also enhance recall of emotionally similar memories but may inhibit recall of emotionally dissimilar information (for example, Isen, 1987). Happy or pleasant feelings are accordingly likely to cue happy or positive associations and memories, whereas fearful feelings will tend to promote fearful or anxious associations. Given the focus here on health care art, an important implication of emotional congruence theory is that patients should tend to perceive, interpret, and have associations with art in ways that match their emotional states or feelings (Ulrich, 1999).

Here, the point cannot be overemphasized that patients experience stress and negatively toned feelings (fear, anxiety, anger, and sadness), and that many suffer acute emotional distress. It can be predicted on the basis of emotional congruence theory that such negative feelings could dispose patients to perceive and interpret certain art styles and subject matter in emotionally matching negatively stressful ways (Ulrich, 1999). A related prediction is that acutely stressed patients could be especially vulnerable to interpreting art as stressful or even frightening when the styles and subject matter are abstract or ambiguous—and can be readily interpreted in widely different ways (Ulrich, 1999). According to emotional congruence theory, a healthy person in good spirits may tend to respond to an abstract or ambiguous painting in an emotionally matching positive manner. The same person could be more prone to reacting negatively to the identical painting, however, when he or she is hospitalized and experiencing strongly negative feelings. The message from emotional congruence theory is that caution should be exercised when considering ambiguous or abstract art for patient spaces or high-stress waiting and treatment areas. It follows that the most prudent "do no harm" course when selecting art for acutely stressed patients is to emphasize works with unambiguously positive subject matter that resists negative interpretations (Ulrich, 1991, 1999; Marberry, 1995).

Research on Preferences for Visual Images

Much research has examined peoples' responses to art and other types of visual images, but the vast majority of studies have measured preferences or liking rather than effects on stress recovery (restoration) and other medical outcomes. Scientifically speaking, the relationship between visual preference responses and restoration/health effects is not well understood. There is limited evidence suggesting that preference appears to play a role in restoration, but the correlation between preference and stress recovery influences may not be consistently high. Notwithstanding this caveat, preference studies are still useful for providing insights about what types of art are most liked by diverse groups of people.

The General Public Prefers Nature Images

Consistent with evolutionary theory, a clear-cut conclusion supported by well over a hundred published preference studies on real visual environments—such as building facades, room interiors, and forests— is that populations from different areas of the world evidence a strong tendency to favor nature scenes over urban or built environments, especially when the latter lack nature content such as foliage and water (Ulrich, 1983, 1993). Consistently preferred types of nature environments include settings with nonturbulent water features, savanna-like or park-like environments with scattered trees and moderate to high depths of field, and distant mountain ranges with low hills and scattered foreground trees (Ulrich, 1983; Patsfall, Feimer, Buhyoff, and Wellman, 1984). Also, cross-national research on scenes with trees has shown that adult groups mostly prefer trees with broad canopies and relatively short bifurcated trunks (Sommer and Summit, 1996; Summit and Sommer, 1999).

These environmental preference findings are echoed by art studies showing that the great majority of adults across different cultures
like realistic or representational nature art (Kettlewell, 1988; Winston and Cupchik, 1992; Wypijewski, 1997). A considerable majority of adults internationally also evidences striking similarity in
disliking abstract art and sculpture (Wypijewski, 1997). Furthermore,
a finding that should be highlighted for its health care implications
is that the greater part of the public considers art aesthetically pleasing if it engenders positive feelings such as happiness and pleasantness. In this regard, a study of a national random sample of adult
Americans found that most people strongly agreed with statements
such as "I only want to look at art that makes me happy" and "art
should be relaxing to look at" (Wypijewski, 1997).

Patient Art Preferences

A limited amount of research on hospital patient art preferences
has yielded findings consistent with those for the nonpatient public. Carpman and Grant (1993) showed a varied collection of pictures to three hundred randomly selected inpatients and asked them
to rate each picture for how much they would like to have it hanging in their hospital room. Results indicated that the hospital inpatients consistently preferred representational nature scenes but
disliked or rejected abstract art.

Hathorn and Ulrich (2001) carried out small-scale preliminary
studies at a university hospital in a major city to assess the health
care art preferences of groups of African Americans and whites. Participants were given binders containing a highly diverse collection
of 676 color pictures of paintings and were asked to rate how appropriate or inappropriate each picture was for display in patient areas.
Consistent with the evolutionary proposition that nature scenes
should elicit positive responses across different groups of people,
findings showed that both blacks and whites rated as very appropriate and preferred representational paintings of nature landscapes
and rural areas (Hathorn and Ulrich, 2001). Irrespective of race or

ethnicity, participants gave especially positive ratings to nature paintings showing spatially open settings in clear, sunny weather, with water features and verdant or healthy green vegetation. As well, paintings of gardens with flowers were consistently rated as highly appropriate and preferred.

The same preliminary studies further suggested that both blacks and whites judged as appropriate figurative artworks that depicted people with clearly positive facial/emotional expressions, who displayed body language and gestures that were caring or friendly (Hathorn and Ulrich, 2001). These findings for figurative art are congruent with the proposition from evolutionary theory that was mentioned earlier; that is, humans have a partly genetic predisposition to respond positively to images of smiling or caring faces.

Art Preferences of Artists and Designers

The art preferences of artists, environmental designers, and people seriously interested in art, however, differ greatly from those of the general public—and the subset of the public who are patients (Ulrich, 1999). In complete contrast with the great majority of the public, artists and experienced art viewers like artworks that are challenging or emotionally provocative (Winston and Cupchik, 1992). Moreover, they *disagree* with the notion that art should produce positive feelings in a broad audience. They further differ from the public in that they tend to like artwork that ranges across a diversity of styles—abstract as well as representational. In sum, many artists and designers enjoy provocative emotional "payoffs" when viewing art, and they like art styles and subject matter that evoke negative reactions in most of the public. This implies that if artists and designers follow their personal aesthetic tastes and knowledge when selecting art for health care settings and fail to involve patient representatives or consult research evidence, they may unwittingly specify art that widely misses the mark of patient preferences and therefore provokes negative reactions (Ulrich, 1999).

Research on Stress-Reducing Effects of Visual Images

In a manner that somewhat parallels findings regarding art preferences of the general public, studies of restorative effects of visual
stimuli have identified representational nature images as tending to
be stress-reducing. These research results are in harmony with evolutionary writings described earlier.

Several studies of nonpatient groups (university students, for
example) have converged in indicating that nature scenes dominated by vegetation, flowers, or water—as compared with the great
majority of built scenes lacking nature—are considerably more
effective in promoting recovery from stress. (For surveys of studies,
see Ulrich, 1999; Parsons and Hartig, 2000.) Nature images need
not be aesthetically superb in order to have stress-reducing effects.
A fine painting of a vista such as the Yosemite Valley would likely
work very well, but even an undistinguished painting of a garden or
lake can produce measurable restoration from stress.

Convincing scientific evidence shows that the restorative effects
of viewing nature are achieved within only three to five minutes as a
combination of positive physiological and emotional/psychological
changes (Ulrich and others, 1991; Parsons and Hartig, 2000). Concerning the first psychological indications of stress recovery, studies
in both laboratories and real environments have consistently found
that viewing nature can promote substantial restoration in less than
five minutes, as is evident, for instance, in blood pressure, heart
activity, muscle tension, and brain electrical activity (Ulrich and
others, 1991; Parsons, 1991). Regarding emotional/psychological
effects, looking at most nature views elevates positive feelings such as
pleasantness and calm and lessens negatively toned emotions such
as anxiety, anger, and dejection (Ulrich, 1979). Furthermore, many
nature scenes effectively sustain positive interest and thus function as
pleasant distractions that may block worrisome, stressful thoughts.
Regarding the positive emotional effects of looking at nature,

Fredrickson and Levenson (1998) have proposed that one key function of positive emotions is to "undo" elevated physiological stress arousal produced by negative feelings—for example, anxiety.

As an example of restoration research in a controlled laboratory setting, 120 nonpatients were first shown a stressful movie and were then randomly assigned to a stress recovery situation that consisted of viewing a videotape (not artwork) either of unspectacular nature settings or of comparatively attractive built environments (Ulrich and others, 1991). Findings from a battery of physiological measures (such as of blood pressure, heart rate, skin conductance, and muscle tension) were consistent in showing that recuperation from stress was faster and more complete when individuals were exposed to the nature rather than built settings. The physiological data further suggested that nature effectively lowered activity in the sympathetic nervous system, which is noteworthy because heightened sympathetic activity is central in stress responses. Finally, self-ratings of feelings indicated that people exposed to the nature settings, in contrast with the built environments, had lower levels of fear and anger and far higher levels of positive emotions (Ulrich and others, 1991).

An example of research that took place in real environments rather than in a laboratory is Hartig's study (1991) of Los Angeles residents who were stressed either because they had just driven in city traffic or because they had performed difficult problem solving tests. His findings were broadly similar to those just described— blood pressure recordings and emotional self-reports together indicated that recovery was appreciably greater when people looked at a nature setting rather than a built environment lacking nature (Hartig, 1991).

Pictures of outstanding architecture can be liked aesthetically, but they appear not to produce restoration as effectively as most nature scenes. Hartig and his colleagues (1996) assigned nonpatient subjects in Sweden to a slide-simulated "walk" through either an attractive area of Stockholm with fine architecture but little nature or through an unspectacular nature area. Findings suggested that looking at nature promoted more relaxation and greater overall emotional well-being than did the viewing of an exceptionally attractive built district.

In the discussion up to this point, restoration or stress recovery has been used in reference to recuperation from excessively high physiological excitement or activity levels, accompanied by negatively toned feelings and thoughts. But restoration is a broader concept that also is relevant to recovery from excessively low excitement or arousal linked with understimulation and boredom (Ulrich and others, 1991). For groups suffering from boredom and underarousal (such as employees with monotonous jobs or many long-term patients in nursing homes), the capacity of visual images to be positively interesting and mildly stimulating over long time periods becomes a key therapeutic issue. Importantly, evidence suggests that representational landscape pictures outperform other categories of visual subject matter when installed for extended periods in isolated and confined work environments where boredom is a problem.

One investigation by Clearwater and Coss (1991) focused on scientists who worked for one year in isolated and confined circumstances in antarctic research stations. The researchers found that nature landscape pictures, both with and without water features, were more effective than other types of subject matter in sustaining interest, preference, and relaxation throughout the year of isolated work. Spatially open nature landscapes proved superior to such pictures as those depicting humans in action or wild animals. In the second study, the investigators displayed a collection of ninety-five pictures of sixteenth- to twentieth-century paintings to volunteers confined in a realistic mock-up of a module for the International Space Station (Clearwater and Coss, 1991). Types of subject matter included nature landscapes, landscapes with prominent buildings, animals in nature settings, close-up pictures of human artifacts, and people engaged in athletic and recreational activities. Findings suggested that in the confined setting of the space station mock-up, people responded most positively to paintings of natural landscapes with high depth of field.

Effects of Viewing Nature on Patient Stress and Other Outcomes

Similar to laboratory findings for stressed nonpatients, a limited amount of research focusing on patients has found that looking at nature images for only a few minutes can promote significant restoration, even in acutely stressed individuals. An investigation by Heerwagen (1990), for example, suggested that stress in a dental clinic was appreciably lower on days when a large nature mural was hung on a wall of the waiting room, in contrast with days when the wall was blank. This conclusion was supported both by heart rate recordings from patients and questionnaire findings. Coss (1990) displayed ceiling-mounted pictures to highly stressed patients lying on gurneys in a presurgical holding room and reported that patients had lower blood pressure when exposed to serene nature photographs than when assigned either a control condition of no picture or beautiful but stimulating pictures, such as a seascape with brisk wind conditions.

Findings from a few studies suggest that visual exposure to real nature not only reduces patient stress but also improves other medical outcomes. An investigation of inpatients recovering from gall bladder surgery found that people with a bedside window view of nature (grove of trees) had more positive postoperative courses than matched patients who were assigned rooms looking out at a brick wall (Ulrich, 1984). Patients with the nature window view had shorter hospital stays, tended to have fewer minor complications, such as persistent nausea, and received far fewer negative comments about their conditions in nurses' notes, such as "patient is upset" or "needs much encouragement." Furthermore, the nature view patients, compared with those with the brick wall window view, experienced less pain, as evidenced by their taking many fewer doses of potent narcotic analgesics (Ulrich, 1984).

Another study evaluated the therapeutic effects of a videotape of scenic nature (forest, flowers, ocean) accompanied by a music soundtrack for burn patients suffering intense pain (Miller, Hick-man, and Lemasters, 1992). The investigators reported that the nature videotape significantly benefited the patients during burn dressing changes by reducing pain intensity and reported anxiety. Although the nature videotape likely played a major role in these important outcome improvements, its specific contribution is unclear because music was also a factor.

Effects of Nature Versus Abstract Images on Outcomes

A study at a university hospital in Sweden investigated whether dis-playing different types of pictures, including abstracts and realistic nature scenes, improved outcomes following heart surgery (Ulrich, Lundén, and Eltinge, 1993). One hundred and sixty heart surgery patients on intensive care units were each assigned to one of six pic-ture interventions: two representational nature scenes (one dominated by water and trees, the other a forest), two types of abstract pictures (one having straight or rectilinear contours, the other curvilinear forms), or two control conditions (either no picture or a white panel). A picture was mounted above the foot of each patient's bed and in the patient's line of vision. Results suggested that patients exposed to the landscape picture with water, trees, and high depth of field experienced less anxiety and suffered less intense pain than patients assigned to any of the other five picture conditions (Ulrich, Lundén, and Eltinge, 1993). A picture of a forest setting with shadowy areas, however, did not significantly improve outcomes, compared with the control conditions.

An unexpected finding in the heart surgery study was that the abstract picture dominated by straight-edged forms worsened out-comes, compared with having no picture at all (Ulrich, Lundén, and Eltinge, 1993; Ulrich, 1999). Several patients assigned this rectilinear abstract picture had distinctly negative reactions when looking at it, necessitating immediate removal of the picture. Despite the fact that none of these patients had any medical history of serious psychological disturbance, the ambiguity of the straight-edged abstract nonetheless evoked aversive emotional reactions and some frightening associations. It is plausible to suggest that such negative reactions can be understood in light of emotional congruence theory. As pointed out earlier, this theory implies that acutely stressed patients, such as those in the heart surgery study, would be vulnerable to interpreting art as stressful or frightening when the styles and subject matter are ambiguous or abstract and can be perceived in widely different ways (Ulrich, 1999). Perhaps the heart surgery patients' stressful feelings tended to mold their interpretations of the ambiguous straight-edged abstract in emotionally matching negative ways.

An earlier small-scale study of psychiatric patients in a Swedish hospital similarly found that patients responded positively to representational nature paintings and prints but reacted negatively to several abstract artworks (Ulrich, 1986, 1991, 1999). The ward was extensively furnished with wall-mounted paintings and prints. In interviews, patients reported having positive feelings and associations with respect to the great majority of nature pictures (for example, a garden or a rural landscape with a farm). By contrast, several individuals expressed negative reactions to abstract artworks in which the content was ambiguous and could be interpreted in multiple ways. Moreover, archival data for the previous fifteen years revealed that patients had physically attacked seven of the paintings and prints (Ulrich, 1986, 1991). Five of them had been attacked more than once and therefore had been placed in storage. The attacks were dramatic actions, given that these patients were considered unaggressive and not at all prone to violence. The attacked artworks, it should be emphasized, consistently displayed abstract styles and ambiguous content. Most of the pictures portrayed disordered, comparatively chaotic arrays of contrasting colors and abstract elements.

Further evidence of the potential for ambiguous or abstract art to have unintended negative effects comes from the well-documented example of a large-scale sculpture installation created as a window view for cancer patients (Ulrich, 1999). The purpose of the sculpture was to create a pleasant and restorative visual distraction for patients. This "Bird Garden" installation contained many bird figures executed in abstract and representational styles. (Although called a "garden," the installation contained no flowers or other nature.) Prominent in the installation were several tall metal sculptures dominated by rectilinear contours and abstract forms, many having pointed or piercing features.

Shortly after the sculpture was installed hospital administrators began to receive anecdotal reports of strong negative reactions by some patients (McLaughlin and others, 1996). In response to these concerns, a questionnaire study was conducted to make possible an evidence-based assessment of the effects of the artworks. Twenty-two percent of the cancer patients reported having an overall negative emotional response to the sculpture garden (Hefferman, Morstatt, Saltzman, and Strunc, 1995). Many found the art installation ambiguous ("doesn't make any sense"), which may explain why some people reacted in strongly negative ways that emotionally matched their distressed feelings as patients with cancer (Ulrich, 1999). Consistent with emotional congruence theory, certain patients interpreted the sculptures, for instance, as frightening predators. Administrators and medical staff members decided that the rate and intensity of negative reactions was too high; accordingly, the art installation was removed for medical reasons.

Finally, Staricoff and her associates (Staricoff and others, 2001) administered a questionnaire to several hundred patients, visitors, and staff members at a London hospital to evaluate an arts program that included paintings, sculpture, and live musical performances. The collection of paintings and sculpture contained many works with representational nature content as well as several abstracts. Findings showed that patients, visitors, and staff members responded quite positively to the visual art collection as a whole, reporting that the paintings and sculpture helped ease their stress levels and distracted them from their worries. Because the questionnaire assessed the overall collection, however, the findings did not permit evaluation of individual artworks or compare responses to the nature with responses to the abstract paintings and sculpture. It is worth noting that patients rated live musical performances as more effective than visual art in distracting them from immediate worries and medical problems (Staricoff and others, 2001).

Evidence-Based Guidelines for Selecting Health Care Art

On the basis of the foregoing discussion of theory and research, this section lists evidence-based guidelines intended to increase the likelihood that the health care art (paintings, prints, and photographs) selected will improve outcomes for stressed patients (Ulrich, 1991; Marberry, 1995; Hathorn and Ulrich, 2001). In view of the limited amount of scientific research currently available, there is no suggestion here that the guidelines are comprehensive or that they encompass in a complete sense all art selection considerations that might affect patient well-being and health.

It is recommended that all the visual art (paintings, prints, and photographs) displayed in patient areas have unambiguously positive subject matter and convey a sense of security or safety. In addition, priority should be given to selecting representational art that depicts the following categories of subject matter:

Waterscapes

- Calm or nonturbulent water, not stormy conditions

Landscapes

- Visual depth or openness in immediate foreground

- Landscapes depicted during warmer seasons when vegetation is verdant and flowers are visible; landscapes conveying bleakness should be avoided

- Scenes with positive cultural artifacts such as barns and older houses

- Landscapes with low hills and distant mountains

Flowers/Gardens

- Flowers that appear healthy and fresh, not wilted or dead

- Types of flowers that are generally familiar to patients, not novel or strange

- Garden scenes with some openness in the immediate foreground

Figurative Art

- Emotionally positive facial expressions

- Relationships among people that are friendly, caring, or nurturing

- Generational and cultural diversity

- People at leisure in places with prominent nature

The following characteristics should usually be avoided when selecting art for stressed patients (Ulrich, 1991; Marberry, 1995; Hathorn and Ulrich, 2001):

- Ambiguity or uncertainty

- Emotionally negative or provocative subject matter

- Surreal qualities

- Closely spaced repeating edges or forms that are optically unstable or appear to move

- Restricted depth or claustrophobic-like qualities

- Close-up animals staring directly at the viewer

- Outdoor scenes with overcast or foreboding weather

Conclusions Concerning the Effect of Visual Art on Medical Outcomes

It is evident from the research survey that scientific knowledge concerning the effect that visual art has on medical outcomes is at an early stage of development. Nonetheless, when findings from the small number of art studies are considered together with those from more numerous investigations based on photographs, videotapes, or real views, the combined evidence is clearly encouraging. That is, the cumulative findings indicate that certain types of psychologically appropriate art and other visual stimuli can evoke positive emotional responses, effectively reduce stress, and improve other outcomes. At the same time, there is increasing evidence that psychologically or emotionally inappropriate art styles or image subject matter can increase patient stress and worsen other outcomes. Accordingly, the overall findings strongly support the conclusion that art selection for health care facilities should be evidence-based.

A reliable finding to emerge from several studies is that certain types of representational nature images can within minutes promote significant improvement in emotional/psychological and physiological measures of patient stress. Another noteworthy finding from different studies is that viewing nature can alleviate pain, as evidenced, for instance, by reduced intake of pain medication. Furthermore, there is mounting evidence that abstract or ambiguous images evoke dislike or other distinctly negative reactions in many patients. Regarding this last point, the discussion has emphasized that designers and medical professionals should exercise caution before displaying ambiguous or emotionally challenging art in patient rooms or other spaces where stress is a problem.

On the basis of the limited scientific knowledge available, the most prudent and effective general approach for selecting art for patients is to feature representational nature images and figurative works showing positive facial expressions and friendly or caring relationships. To further increase the likelihood that art will beneficially affect the great majority of patients and visitors, it is suggested that *all* works display unambiguously positive subject matter that resists negative interpretations, even by acutely stressed individuals. Finally, providing patients with an opportunity to choose their own art (an art cart program, for example) should enhance personal control and help ensure that images promote improved outcomes (Ulrich, 1991; Marberry, 1995).

In conclusion, the research discussed in this chapter implies that visual artwork in health care facilities is no mere luxury or unimportant embellishment. To the contrary, findings increasingly support the notion that the evidence-based selection of emotionally appropriate art contributes an important environmental dimension to patient care—one that lessens patient stress and improves other medical outcomes.

Healing, Music, and the Arts

Planetree's emphasis on the arts was inspired by the healing temples of ancient Greece. Here, as in many other cultures throughout the world, the arts have been used in healing rituals to revitalize patients' inner resources, restore their will to survive, and rekindle the joy of living. Music has been used throughout the centuries to calm and soothe or enliven and invigorate. And such expressive arts as painting and working with clay offer patients the opportunity to give form to their emotions. In the Planetree model, the arts have been described as inspiration for the mind, language for the emotions, and balm for the soul. In addition, the visual arts, music, storytelling, poetry, humor, and other expressive arts can all play a vital role in creating a healing environment for patients and their families, as well as providing a positive working environment for the staff.

While many studies document the physiological effects of the arts on health and healing, many hospitals choose to include a variety of arts simply for their usefulness as "positive distractions," offering a diversion from anxiety, discomfort, and loneliness. Whereas art therapy uses the arts, in conjunction with counseling skills, as a therapeutic technique, the purpose of Planetree arts programs is simply to bring the experience of the arts to patients and their families. This experience can offer a respite from the intensity of illness and the anxiety of hospitalization. The arts can also diminish boredom and provide a space for reflection and inspiration.

An arts program need not be expensive. Many operate primarily with volunteers and donated equipment. Many hospitals find that community groups, local art associations, and volunteers are willing to donate time and resources to create and maintain an active arts program. The arts program at the first Planetree site began with a weekly movie night and a few donated audiotapes and cassette players for patients. After its initial success, the program was expanded.

Arts programs vary at Planetree sites. Some examples include the following:

• *Shands at AGH.* A community hospital in Gainesville, Florida, Shands has created an extensive Arts in Healing program. In addition to many volunteers, the program has three artists-in-residence, who receive small stipends and spend four to eight hours per week at the hospital. These artists-in-residence, including an oral historian, a visual artist, and a musician, provide a visible artistic presence and serve as mentors for volunteers.

The oral historian works with patients to help them tell their stories, which she writes down for the patients or families to keep. When a patient dies, many family members thank her for this meaningful keepsake.

The visual artist paints small pastel portraits of patients or family members throughout the hospital. When a patient in the emergency department is hostile or disruptive, staff members call the artist, who provides a calming diversion for the patient by painting a portrait. The patient is then given the portrait as a gift. The visual artist has also attended the reunion of babies from the neonatal ICU, to create a collage of the children's handprints to offer hope to parents with babies currently in the NICU.

The musical artist-in-residence plays the piano and guitar throughout the hospital and serves as a mentor for the arts volunteers. Staff members in the NICU have reported that harp music, played by one of the volunteers, has a calming effect on the babies.

In addition to the artists in residence, Shands at AGH has approximately seventy-five arts volunteers, including many University of Florida premedical students who are members of the American Medical Student Association. Other students from the university volunteer as strolling musicians or they assist patients with bedside arts projects. Volunteer orientations are held on campus to encourage participation. The summer "volunteen" program for high school students has been so successful that some students have been turned away until more opportunities for volunteens can be created.

Volunteers who do not play instruments work with the art carts to encourage patients to express themselves through art activities. Families in the surgical waiting areas are encouraged to use the art supplies to make get well cards to present to the patients immediately after surgery.

Shands at AGH has linked with the community by hosting monthly meetings of the "clown alley." In exchange, local clowns, some professionally trained, volunteer at the hospital to entertain patients and teach classes in the community for others interested in clowning. Humor carts, filled with clown noses, puppets, and silly stickers, encourage patients and family members to join the fun. "Joy Jars," filled with candy, games, and stickers, are available on the oncology unit as a resource for nurses who may need to cheer up cancer patients.

Several medical-surgical units have CD players so that patients can listen to their own CDs or those available from the hospital's collection. Music students at the University of Florida, preparing for their senior recitals, are encouraged to practice in front of an audience of patients and families in the hospital lobby.

The value of the Arts in Healing program at Shands at AGH was voiced by a surgical ICU patient recovering from bypass surgery. After being visited by a violinist, a clown, and a pet therapy dog, he commented, "I didn't know you could have this much fun in a hospital."

• *Mid-Columbia Medical Center.* Mid-Columbia Medical Center (MCMC) in The Dalles, Oregon, involved school children from the community in painting a forty-four-foot mural depicting life on the Oregon Trail, which reflects the local history. In addition, children from the hospital's day care center periodically visit the hospital to sing.

MCMC also has approximately fifty adult arts volunteers. Some volunteers help with the "art cart," which consists of a book of photographs of the artwork available, enabling patients to select the artwork for their own rooms. The "art cart" enables patients to personalize the space or find images that they believe are healing.

Many musicians and local choirs volunteer to give performances in the atrium for patients, families, and staff members. The atrium was designed to accommodate forty to fifty people, and balconies on each patient floor enable those less mobile to hear the music. Local piano teachers are invited to hold recitals in the atrium.

At MCMC's cancer center, artwork in the barrel vault ceiling above the simulator and linear accelerator was designed to change as light in the room changes. One scene creates the image of lying under a blossoming cherry tree. Watching the artwork change with the light provides a distraction for patients undergoing the often anxiety-filled experience of a radiation procedure.

MCMC's Celilo Center, named for the sacred Native American fishing grounds, includes a water feature with eleven different petroglyphs, or rock carvings, representing healing and spiritual images. Developed in conjunction with local historians and a Native American shaman, the water feature is reminiscent of the waterfalls that are a familiar part of the landscape in the Columbia River gorge. The eleven petroglyphs, which cannot be seen from any one place at the Celilo Center, create a sense of discovery for patients and family members who may need to return repeatedly for ongoing cancer treatments.

One physician, who specializes in stress management, invites patients, families, and staff members to participate in drumming circles. A local guitarist, Michael Stillwater, writes and records music for patients, who are then given the tape as a gift. A music thanatologist, trained in the Chalice of Repose tradition, holds vigils for dying patients, playing music tailored to the patients' physiological and emotional changes.

- *Griffin Hospital.* This hospital in Derby, Connecticut, brings music into the parking lot, where patients and visitors are greeted by softly playing background music as soon as they leave their cars. Once inside the hospital, professional musicians provide music seven days a week, three or four times a day. The musicians have been selected for their talent as well as for their appreciation of the role that music can play in healing. They are paid a small fee to cover their travel.

The hospital has five pianos, one in the lobby and the others on patient floors, bringing the music directly to the patients, families, and staff. In addition to piano, some musicians play guitar, banjo, and harmonica. Griffin's Arts and Entertainment Program includes fifty-five active participants, who bring music to a variety of settings. A guitarist is scheduled to play in the out-patient laboratory, where patients may be anxious about having their blood drawn. Music is often available to patients during special procedures, such as when they receive chemotherapy or blood transfusions. Patients from the psychiatric unit have been especially appreciative of the music.

The musicians and arts volunteers provide approximately 120 to 140 hours of arts and entertainment every month. Storytelling for children in the Health Resource Center has been well attended. The magician, dressed in a tuxedo and red bow tie, performs card tricks at the bedside. Arts and crafts are brought to the patients' rooms, where they can make wreaths or paint ceramic cups that are given to them as gifts.

Artwork on the walls throughout the hospital was selected to be life-enhancing. Peaceful scenes of flowers, trails, and waterfalls add to the healing environment.

• *Longmont United Hospital.* In addition to visual art and music, Longmont United Hospital in Longmont, Colorado, has developed a clown program in the tradition of the physician clown, Patch Adams. Several years ago, a hospital volunteer, who had extensive training as a clown, created the Clown College for interested staff members and volunteers. Over twenty staff members from a variety of departments, as well as volunteers, are now graduates of Clown College. Once a week, in full clown regalia, they volunteer for "Clown Rounds," visiting patients and greeting visitors in the lobby. They entertain by pulling playful toys from their box of tricks (in reality, a box of Trix, the cereal) and by handing out "brownies" (the letter "e" cut from brown paper). Their silly antics amuse and delight the young and old—particularly some elderly patients, who have few visitors and are often lonely.

• *Stratton VA Medical Center.* Stratton VA Medical Center in Albany, New York, receives a donation that enables it to bring in the professional group Clowns on Rounds to entertain patients and families.

• *Albert Einstein Medical Center.* Philadelphia's Albert Einstein Medical Center provides music and massage for its cardiac catheterization patients. Patients are encouraged to bring their favorite music or listen to a CD from the hospital's collection.

• *Beth Israel Medical Center.* The Juilliard School of Music in New York gives volunteer performances once a month at Beth Israel Medical Center in Manhattan.

• *Forum Health's Trumbull Memorial Hospital.* Trumbull Memorial Hospital in Warren, Ohio, has an extensive arts program, including rotating art exhibits by local artists. A poetry corner displays the whimsical picture poems of local poet Kenneth Patchen. A healing garden provides an ideal setting for performances by local musicians.

Some Planetree hospitals have VCRs in each patient room. Others offer the Care Channel, a closed-circuit channel offering photographs of nature with the music of Susan Maser and Dallas Smith. New technology is being developed to enable patients to have greater accessibility to the arts.

The arts are an integral part of people's lives. And illness and hospitalization is a time when the arts may be most needed to nurture patients' healing.

References

Appleton, J. *The Experience of Landscape.* London: Wiley, 1975.

Bower, G. "Mood and Memory." *American Psychologist,* 1981, *36,* 129–148.

Carpman, J. R., and Grant, M. A. *Design That Cares: Planning Health Facilities for Patients and Visitors.* (2nd. ed.) Chicago: American Hospital Publishing, 1993.

Clearwater, Y. A., and Coss, R. G. "Functional Aesthetics to Enhance Well-Being in Isolated and Confined Settings." In A. A. Harrison, Y. A. Clearwater, and C. McKay (eds.), *From Antarctica to Outer Space: Life in Isolation and Confinement.* New York: Springer-Verlag, 1991.

Coss, R. G. "The Ethological Command in Art." *Leonardo,* 1968, *1,* 273–287.

Coss, R. G. "Picture Perception and Patient Stress: A Study of Anxiety Reduction and Postoperative Stability." Unpublished paper, Department of Psychology, University of California, Davis, 1990.

Coss, R. G. "The Role of Evolved Perceptual Biases in Art and Design." In E. Voland, K. Grammer, and A. Heschl (eds.), *Evolutionary Aesthetics: On the Evolution of Aesthetic Value Judgments.* Cambridge, Mass.: MIT Press, forthcoming.

Darwin, C. *The Expression of Emotions in Man and Animals.* Chicago: University of Chicago Press, 1965. (Originally published 1872.)

Easterbrook, M. A., Kisilevsky, B. S., Hains, S. M., and Muir, D. W. "Faceness or Complexity: Evidence from Newborn Visual Tracking of Face-Like Stimuli." *Infant Behavior and Development,* 1999, *22,* 17–35.

Ekman, P., Friesen, W. V., and Ellsworth, P. C. *Emotion in the Human Face*. New York: Pergamon Press, 1972.

Fredrickson, B. L., and Levenson, R. W. "Positive Emotions Speed Recovery from the Cardiovascular Sequelae of Negative Emotions." *Cognition and Emotion*, 1998, *12*, 191–220.

Friedrich, M. J. "The Healing Arts." *JAMA*, May 19, 1999, 1779–1781.

Hathorn, K., and Ulrich, R. S. "The Therapeutic Art Program of Northwestern Memorial Hospital." In *Creating Environments That Heal: Proceedings of the Symposium on Healthcare Design* (CD-Rom). Imark Communications, in association with the Center for Health Design, 2001. [www.hcaredesign.com].

Hartig, T. "Testing Restorative Environments Theory." Unpublished doctoral dissertation, Program in Social Ecology, University of California Press, Irvine, 1991.

Hartig, T., and others. "Environmental Influences on Psychological Restoration." *Scandinavian Journal of Psychology*, 1996, *37*, 378–393.

Heerwagen, J. "The Psychological Aspects of Windows and Window Design." In K. H. Anthony, J. Choi, and B. Orland (eds.), *Proceedings of the Twenty-First Annual Conference of the Environmental Design Research Association*. Oklahoma City: Environmental Design Research Association, 1990.

Hefferman, M. L., Morstatt, M., Saltzman, K., and Strunc, L. "A Room with a View Art Survey: The Bird Garden at Duke University Hospital." Unpublished research report, Cultural Services Program and Management Fellows Program, Duke University Medical Center, Durham, N.C., 1995.

Isen, A. "Positive Affect, Cognitive Processes, and Social Behavior." In L. Berkowitz (ed.), *Advances in Experimental Social Psychology*. Orlando, Fla.: Academic Press, 1987.

Johnson, M. H., Dziurawiec, S., Ellis, H., and Morton, J. "Newborns' Preferential Tracking of Face-Like Stimuli and Its Subsequent Decline." *Cognition*, 1991, *40*, 1–19.

Kaplan, R., and Kaplan, S. *The Experience of Nature*. New York: Cambridge University Press, 1989.

Kendler, K. S., Karkowski, L. M., and Prescott, C. A. "Fears and Phobias: Reliability and Heritability." *Psychological Medicine*, 1999, *29*, 539–553.

Kettlewell, N. "An Examination of Preferences for Subject Matter in Art." *Empirical Studies of the Arts*, 1988, 6, 59–65.

Marberry, S. O. (ed.). *Innovations in Healthcare Design*. New York: Van Nostrand Reinhold, 1995.

Martin, C. "Let Me Through—I'm an Arts Practitioner!" *The Lancet*, Apr. 24, 1999, p. 1451.

McLaughlin, J., and others. "Duke University's Bird Garden." In *Proceedings of the 1996 Annual Conference of the Society for the Arts in Healthcare*. Durham, N.C.: Durham Arts Council and Duke University Medical Center, 1996.

Miller, A. C., Hickman, L. C., and Lemasters, G. K. "A Distraction Technique for Control of Burn Pain." *Journal of Burn Care and Rehabilitation*, 1992, *13*, 576–580.

Niedenthal, P. M., Setterlund, M. B., and Jones, D. E. "Emotional Organization of Perceptual Memory." In P. M. Niedenthal and S. Kitayama (eds.), *The Heart's Eye: Emotional Influences in Perception and Attention*. Orlando, Fla.: Academic Press, 1994.

Nightingale, F.. *Notes on Nursing*. New York: Dover, 1969. (Originally published 1860.)

Öhman, A. "Face the Beast and Fear the Face: Animal and Social Fears as Prototypes for Evolutionary Analyses of Emotion." *Psychophysiology*, 1986, *23*, 123–145.

Orians, G. H. "An Ecological and Evolutionary Approach to Landscape Aesthetics." In E. C. Penning-Rowsell and D. Lowenthal (eds.), *Meanings and Values in Landscape*. London: Allen and Unwin, 1986.

Parsons, R. "Recovery from Stress During Exposure to Videotaped Outdoor Environments." Doctoral dissertation, Department of Psychology, University of Arizona Press, Tucson, 1991.

Parsons, R. and Hartig, T. "Environmental Psychophysiology." In J. T. Cacioppo, L. G. Tassinary, and G. Berntson (eds.), *Handbook of Psychophysiology*. New York: Cambridge University Press, 2000.

Patsfall, M. R., Feimer, N. R., Buhyoff, G. J., and Wellman, J. D. "The Prediction of Scenic Beauty from Landscape Content and Composition." *Journal of Environmental Psychology*, 1984, *4*, 7–26.

Singer, J. A., and Salovey, P. "Mood and Memory: Evaluating the Network Theory of Affect." *Clinical Psychology Review*, 1988, *8*, 211–251.

Sommer, R., and Summit, J. "Cross-National Rankings of Tree Shape." *Ecological Psychology*, 1996, *8*, 327–341.

Staricoff, R. S., and others. "A Study of the Effects of the Visual and Performing Arts in Healthcare." *Hospital Development*, June 2001, pp. 25–28.

Summit, J., and Sommer, R. "Further Studies of Preferred Tree Shapes." *Environment and Behavior*, 1999, *31*, 550–576.

Ulrich, R. S. "Visual Landscapes and Psychological Well-Being." *Landscape Research*, 1979, 4(1), 17–23.

Ulrich, R. S. "Aesthetic and Affective Response to Natural Environment." In I. Altman and J. F. Wohlwill (eds.), *Human Behavior and the Environment, Vol. 6: Behavior and the Natural Environment*. New York: Plenum, 1983.

Ulrich, R. S. "View Through a Window May Influence Recovery from Surgery." *Science*, 1984, *224*, 420–421.

Ulrich, R. S. "Effects of Hospital Environments on Patient Well-Being." *Research Report from the Department of Psychiatry and Behavioural Medicine, University of Trondheim, Norway*, 1986, 9(55), 1–13.

Ulrich, R. S. "Effects of Health Facility Interior Design on Wellness: Theory and Recent Scientific Research." *Journal of Health Care Design*, 1991, *3*, 97–109. (Reprinted in S. O. Marberry [ed.], *Innovations in Healthcare Design*. New York: Van Nostrand Reinhold, 1995.)

Ulrich, R. S. "Biophilia, Biophobia, and Natural Landscapes." In S. A. Kellert and E. O. Wilson (eds.), *The Biophilia Hypothesis*. Washington, D.C.: Island Press/Shearwater, 1993.

Ulrich, R. S. "Effects of Gardens on Health Outcomes: Theory and Research." In C. C. Marcus and M. Barnes (eds.), *Healing Gardens: Therapeutic Benefits and Design Recommendations*. New York: Wiley, 1999.

Ulrich, R. S. "Communicating with the Healthcare Community." In C. A. Shoemaker (ed.), *Bringing People and Plants Together for Health and Well-Being*. Ames: Iowa State University Press, 2002.

Ulrich, R. S., Lundén, O., and Eltinge, J. L. "Effects of Exposure to Nature and Abstract Pictures on Patients Recovering from Heart Surgery." Paper presented at the thirty-third meeting of the Society for Psychophysiological Research, Rottach-Egern, Germany, 1993. (Abstract published in *Psychophysiology*, 1993, *30* (supp. 1), 7.)

Ulrich, R. S., and others. "Stress Recovery During Exposure to Natural and Urban Environments." *Journal of Environmental Psychology*, 1991, *11*, 201–230.

Ulrich, R. S., and Parsons, R. "Influences of Passive Experiences with Plants on Individual Well-Being and Health." In D. Relf (ed.), *The Role of Horticulture in Human Well-Being and Social Development*. Portland, Oreg.: Timber Press, 1992.

Wilson, E. O. *Biophilia*. Cambridge, Mass.: Harvard University Press, 1984.

Winston, A. S., and Cupchik, G. C. "The Evaluation of High Art and Popular Art by Naive and Experienced Viewers." *Visual Arts Research*, 1992, *18*, 1–14.

Wypijewski, J. (ed.). *Painting by the Numbers: Komar and Melamid's Scientific Guide To Art*. New York: Farrar, Straus & Giroux, 1997.

8

Integrating Complementary and Alternative Practices into Conventional Care

David Katz

H istorically, the Planetree model has advocated for patient choice and the availability of time-honored approaches to health care in combination with the best practices offered by conventional Western medicine. Over the last two decades, many Planetree hospitals have incorporated a variety of treatment modalities in response to patient interest. This interest has continued to grow throughout the Western world, fueling a multibillion-dollar complementary and alternative medicine movement, both within and outside the mainstream health care industry.

Definition of Complementary and Alternative Medicine

Complementary and Alternative Medicine (CAM) is one among the numerous designations for diverse medical practices not routinely taught to M.D. candidates in medical school, and neither is it incorporated into conventional medical practice. Each of the terms applied to such practices is limited or objectionable in some way. *Alternative* implies both that such practices are defined by what they are not and that they are exclusive of conventional medical care. *Complementary* implies that such practices are supplemental to *mainstream* medicine. The inconsistency in suggesting that such practices are both alternative and complementary to conventional care has been noted (Druss and Rosenheck, 1999; Katz, 1999). Despite its shortcomings, CAM is the most widely used appellation.

Whatever term is applied, CAM practices encompass a broad range of approaches to health care that include naturopathic medicine, chiropractic, traditional Chinese medicine, acupuncture, mind-body medicine, homeopathy, massage, and many others. Traits widely shared by CAM modalities include an emphasis on the individualization of care, the devotion of time and attention to each patient, a reliance on or faith in the healing powers of the body, and nature. Other than these prevailing characteristics, CAM is in fact an extremely heterogeneous array of practices, ranging from those well supported by scientific evidence to those that defy any plausible scientific explanation, and delivered by providers of widely diverse training and credentials (Katz and others, 2002). Some self-professed CAM practitioners have no formal training and are subject to no formal credentialing. At the other extreme, naturopathic physicians require the same four years of postgraduate training for their N.D. degree as M.D.s do for theirs. The naturopathic scope of practice is regulated by the states.

Some of the distinctions among medical disciplines are captured in their names. Conventional medicine is known as *allopathic medicine*, in which *allo* means different from and *path* refers to disease. The mainstay of allopathic therapy is to "attack" disease states with therapies that are unrelated to the condition being treated. In contrast, *homeopathic* medicine relies on treatments considered similar to (*homeo*) the symptoms being addressed, with the belief that the body will eradicate the disease by responding to the remedy. *Naturopathic* medicine obviously relies on natural treatments in its approach to treatment and healing.

Epidemiology and the Population Significance of CAM

Interest in and use of CAM has experienced a dramatic increase in recent years. Approximately eighty-three million people in the United States (42 percent of the adult population) have reported the use of at least one alternative therapy, with one in two people between the ages of thirty-five and forty-nine using one or more alternative therapies (U.S. Department of Health and Human Services, 1991). Visits to alternative therapy practitioners in 1997 exceeded visits to all primary care physicians by 243 million, with the majority seeking alternative treatment for chronic diseases, syndromes, or pain. An increasing percentage of people seek help from an alternative practitioner while being concurrently treated by an allopathic physician—a rise from 8.3 percent in 1990 to 13.7 percent in 1997 (Eisenberg and others, 1998).

Particularly revealing about the popularity of alternative treatments is the fact that the magnitude of the demand for these therapies continues to rise despite the lack of insurance coverage for such services. Americans spent an estimated $21.2 billion out of pocket for visits to alternative providers in 1997, an increase of 45 percent from 1990. The majority—58 percent—of those surveyed who used alternative therapies did so for disease prevention, whereas 42 percent used such services for actual medical problems. The use of alternative therapies is more prevalent among white, female, better-educated, higher-income (over $50,000 per year) populations (Eisenberg and others, 1998). Although the use of CAM is greatest among people aged thirty to forty-nine years, use among elderly patients—those over sixty-five years of age—is on the rise (currently reported at 39.1 percent) and is likely to increase with the growing incidence of chronic illnesses as populations age. The use of CAM has been found to be especially high in patients with Alzheimer's disease, multiple sclerosis, rheumatic diseases, cancer, AIDS, back problems, anxiety, headaches, and chronic pain (Astin and others, 1998).

Predictors of alternative health care use include poorer health status, a holistic philosophical orientation to health and life, a chronic health condition, classification in a cultural group identifiable by its commitment to environmentalism or its commitment to feminism, and its interest in spirituality and personal growth psychology (Astin and others, 1998). Although research findings vary somewhat, all cite the following reasons people use CAM: dissatisfaction with the ability of conventional medicine to adequately treat chronic illnesses, a desire to avoid the harmful side effects of traditional medicine and treatments, an interest in and greater knowledge of how nutritional, emotional, and lifestyle factors affect health, and a broader focus on disease prevention and overall health (Eisenberg and others, 1998; Astin and others, 1998).

Thus, access to CAM modalities affords patients a greater opportunity to obtain care that is consistent with their beliefs and preferences. The availability of CAM treatments may therefore be considered an important means of patient empowerment. In this way, the provision of CAM options, and a patient-centered approach to care, may be seen as fundamentally interrelated. Given the popularity of CAM in the United States today, one might argue that most patients cannot be fully empowered in their health care decision making without having reasonable access to certain CAM therapies.

Despite the significant increase in the use of alternative therapies over recent years, less than 40 percent of alternative medicine users disclose such information to their primary care provider, which reveals an important disconnect between patients' preferences and their willingness to share these views with their doctors (Eisenberg and others, 1993, 1998; Astin and others, 1998; Elder, Gillchrist, and Minz, 1997; Feldman, 1990; McKee, 1988; Mitchell, 1993; Perelson, 1996). This important deficiency in physician-patient communication (Elder, Gillchrist, and Minz, 1997; Feldman, 1990; McKee, 1988; Rao and others, 1999) may reflect patient dissatisfaction with the conventional medical system (Astin and others, 1998; Perelson, 1996), distrust, or simply an accurate assessment of their physician's level of interest.

There is widespread reticence about, if not outright opposition to, CAM practices among allopathic physicians. Those most opposed to the use of CAM argue that alternative therapists do not have the extensive knowledge that is required to diagnose an illness properly, and they often cite the lack of evidence of the efficacy of CAM (Astin and others, 1998). The latter is the most heatedly debated among proponents of traditional medicine. But the claim that conventional medicine is science that is supported by evidence is not always accurate. The Office of Technology Assessment of the U.S. Congress has estimated that fewer than 30 percent of the procedures currently used in conventional medicine have been rigorously tested (Relman and Weil, 1999). One reason why most alternative therapies are not evidence-based is that the majority were introduced prior to the advent of the randomized controlled clinical trial (RCT). Such limitations are evident in conventional medicine as well; however, they are often overlooked because of the apparent or established effectiveness of a particular treatment. The common and accepted use of antithrombotic agents for cardiovascular diseases and their complications (myocardial infarction, stroke, and pulmonary embolism) supports this contention. Three of the agents prescribed by allopathic physicians for millions of patients every day—warfarin, aspirin, and heparin—were introduced prior to the era of randomized clinical trials and therefore had not been exposed to the rigorous research standards in effect today (Dalen, 1998). Few physicians would consider these drugs unconventional treatments, despite the fact that they were not put through RCTs at the time they were introduced. Conversely, many CAM interventions are indeed supported by methodologically rigorous trials (Katz and others, 2002). Disparities in evidence between conventional and CAM practices do exist—and are likely to persist—because of great discrepancies in the availability of funds to support definitive clinical trials.

With patients increasingly interested in CAM and conventional practitioners widely reticent, a system of unintegrated or, worse, disintegrated health care prevails in the United States. Many conventional physicians actively discourage the use of CAM wholesale, without considering the differences in modalities or practitioners—or the potential value of CAM treatments. Practitioners of CAM may be just as apt to discourage the use of conventional medicine, citing its reliance on dangerous drugs and invasive procedures, its failure to respect the healing powers of Nature, and its lack of compassion and patient-centeredness.

The patient under such conditions is left in a precarious position. Those seeking both conventional care and CAM are likely to receive conflicting advice and to lack the expertise required to make prudent reconciliation between the two. Those choosing to follow both sets of advice may be subject to dangerous interactions that neither half of the care system knows about. Those avoiding a possible conflict by limiting their selection to just one medical discipline may be losing important benefits offered by others, with resultant deficiencies in care. The patient with a chronic health problem for which conventional treatment is ineffective may be left to seek aimlessly among a wide array of therapies, with no place to go for expert guidance that considers all of the options. The costs of such possibly aimless care are likely to be high in both human suffering and dollars, with patients choosing therapies that may be futile, causing them to potentially lose hope and causing insurers to continue to resist including CAM modalities among covered benefits.

Thus, even as CAM in the U.S. health care system is known to be widely and increasingly popular among the public (Eisenberg and others, 1998; Harris and Rees, 2000; Kessler and others, 2001), resistance to the proliferation of CAM among conventionally trained practitioners persists (Marcus, 2001; Beyerstein, 2001; Sampson, 2001; Angell and Kassirer, 1998). Health insurers, although uncertain as to the potential costs and benefits, are subject to increasing pressures to reimburse for various CAM practices (Pelletier, Marie,

Krasner, and Haskell, 1997; Pelletier, Astin, and Haskell, 1999). These tensions and incompatibilities constitute a challenge and threat to patient-centered, holistic approaches to care.

Integrative Medicine

Patient empowerment is one of the dominant principles and trends in modern health care, but there are others. The popularity of CAM is itself an important trend, as is interest in natural therapies and holism. The importance of evidence as the basis for therapies and decisions is an increasingly salient feature in medical education and practice. Finally, the advent of managed care has resulted in increasing attention to the cost-effectiveness of medical interventions.

The confluence of these trends represents the context in which CAM and conventional medicine must coexist. To date, the outpatient setting, where patient autonomy is far greater and regulation of practice is less strict, is where CAM has flourished. With few but noteworthy exceptions, such as the cardiac surgery program at Columbia Presbyterian Medical Center in New York City (Oz, 2002; Okvat, Oz, Ting, and Namerow, 2002), the inpatient setting has been largely inhospitable to CAM thus far. Hospital care is particularly dominated by concerns for evidence-based practice, as well as the stipulations of insurers. Despite this, hospitals are increasingly tempted to address the public's interest in CAM by making some of the most clearly benign therapies, such as massage, available (Hemphill and Kemp, 2000). Such gestures may enhance patient satisfaction and are thus laudable. However, they generally leave control over fundamental aspects of care entirely in the hands of the conventional medical staff.

Efforts to align the interest patients have in alternative care with the practices and procedures of allopathic medicine have resulted in the emergence of *integrative medicine*. As the name implies, this approach to care encompasses both conventional medicine and CAM. However, beyond the name, much of what integrative medicine is—or should be—about is open to interpretation. Andrew Weil, at the University of Arizona, is widely credited with coining the term *integrative medicine*, and he runs a program in which conventional physicians receive supplemental training in CAM disciplines and natural medicine. At other sites, centers are developed in which CAM and conventional practitioners occupy adjacent offices, and refer patients back and forth.

Perhaps the ultimate expression of integrative care is when practitioners from both CAM and conventional medicine make their recommendations available to patients, who can then choose, with expert guidance and support, from a wider array of options. Although few and far between thus far, such models do exist, and they appear likely to proliferate.

The advantages of integrative care, in which diverse practitioners collaborate, are compelling. The traditional wall of silence between CAM and allopathic practice is overcome, thereby avoiding the risk of adverse interactions or gaps in care. Interaction in the care of a patient can help practitioners learn about one another in a manner conducive to more productive collaborations over time. Rather than relying on the limited expertise in all of medicine that any one individual can attain, physicians can take a collaborative approach to care, which provides the patient with access to practitioners who have complementary knowledge and expertise. Because training, credentials, and legitimacy of practice vary widely across the expanse of CAM, and because proficiency varies among conventionally trained physicians, direct communication among practitioners can also help patients identify the most competent, credible, and suitable providers.

As one example of an integrative care model that embraces these principles, the Integrative Medicine Center (IMC) at Griffin Hospital in Derby, Connecticut, offers outpatient care that is fully consensus-based. The IMC is codirected by an allopathic physician and a naturopathic physician. Patients, either self- or physician-referred, are evaluated sequentially by a conventionally trained

medical provider and by a naturopathic physician. Each such evaluation terminates with a consensus conference, in which the
providers from both disciplines review with the patient the array of
treatment options. The IMC is supported by a panel of CAM
providers throughout the state of Connecticut, to whom patients
may be referred for specialized therapies. Among the services the
IMC provides is an evaluation of the credentials and practice history of these practitioners, thereby helping patients find the most
reputable practitioners.

Other models of integrative medicine around the country have
addressed integration in a variety of ways. At Celilo, the new cancer treatment facility at Mid-Columbia Medical Center in The
Dalles, Oregon, radiation therapy and chemotherapy are offered in
conjunction with an array of CAM services. The spa-like setting
includes a meditation garden, saunas, Jacuzzi tubs, and steam rooms.
Staff massage therapists provide pre- and posttreatment massages to
both patients and their waiting family members. Acupuncture is an
important tool that is used to assist in nausea and pain control.
Visualization instruction is provided to elicit the power of the
patient's mind to combat his or her cancer. Humorous videotapes
are available for viewing during treatment sessions. This truly integrative center has far exceeded the initial volume projections, drawing patients from as far away as Portland, Oregon, despite its larger
medical centers. Clearly, patients are willing to travel in order to
access care in a more holistic setting.

The case for integrative medicine at this juncture in the evolution of health care is compelling. Given the clear and growing interest of patients in CAM, a system of care that fails to address CAM
simply cannot be truly patient-centered. Patient-centeredness in
care, the very principle to which the Planetree model is dedicated,
can and should guide medical practices. Patient empowerment and
autonomy, however, should not be at the expense of science and
evidence, and thus wholesale endorsement of CAM in conventional medical institutions is equally inappropriate.

Integrative medicine offers the promise of reconciliation between patient autonomy and interest in CAM with the prevailing conventions of health care. The ultimate goal of integrative care should be to make the widest array of appropriate options available to patients so that they may choose care that feels right for them. Appropriateness should be predicated on fundamental considerations that pertain equally to conventional and CAM practice: treatment safety and treatment effectiveness. Treatment safety and treatment effectiveness must, in turn, be interpreted in light of the available evidence.

The ultimate goal in the evolution of integrative care should be the blurring of boundaries between conventional care and CAM. Both disciplines should be subject to rigorous scientific inquiry so that interventions that work are systematically distinguished from those that don't. Safety should not be assumed in either case but should similarly be derived from rigorous evaluation.

Although the importance of scientific evidence in modern medicine is indisputable, its application is often questionable. Evidence simply does not exist to indicate the best treatment(s) for many chronic conditions and syndromes. Under such circumstances, practitioners who choose to view evidence as the sole basis for medical decisions have nothing to offer. However, evidence could be a tool at the clinicians' disposal rather than the bars of a cage (Katz, 2001). Where strong evidence in support of a particular therapy exists, that therapy should be recommended in preference to others. The less clear it is as to which might be the "right" treatment choice, the more important it is to work down a hierarchy of evidence, considering safety, effectiveness, alternatives, and the evidence supporting each. For many conditions, such as chronic fatigue syndrome or fibromyalgia, a definitive therapy does not exist, and the best available treatments are those likely to be safe—and possibly effective. Access to CAM modalities greatly broadens patient options at this end of the evidence hierarchy, where options are generally most needed.

Many CAM modalities are now well-established aspects of the outpatient health care landscape in the United States. Among these are chiropractic, acupuncture, and mind-body interventions such as meditation, massage therapy, and nutritional supplements (Kessler and others, 2001). Some of these same modalities are available in the hospital setting, although this trend is as yet nascent. Any effort to incorporate CAM practices into conventional care will likely proceed from the more evidence-based, or at least time-honored, CAM modalities, expanding from the outpatient to the inpatient setting.

The ultimate advantages of integrative medicine pertain to both settings. Although inpatient applications are more challenging, many Planetree hospitals have found innovative ways to incorporate these options. For example, at Longmont United Hospital in Longmont, Colorado, every new mother on the maternity unit receives a therapeutic massage following delivery. In order to cover the expense without charging patients, the staff has scrutinized expenditures on the unit, cutting out such things as the traditional "goodie bags" of diapers, powder, and other items, in favor of the massage sessions. Patient satisfaction on the unit has soared, with many patients citing the massage as the most positive aspect of their stay.

Aromatherapy has also made its way into a growing number of inpatient settings, particularly on behavioral health units. Nursing staff members on Griffin Hospital's inpatient psychiatric unit who are trained in aromatherapy employ a variety of scents, distributed via atomizers, to enhance the moods of patients. Studies conducted by the staff on the unit have found that in 90 percent of patients with insomnia, the aroma of lavender has been effective in improving sleep. Sage oil, used for patients with anxiety, effected a 48 percent decrease in scores on the Hamilton Scale, and bergamot oil, used for depressed patients, effected a 45 percent decrease in scores on the Beck Depression scale (M. Schwartz, personal communication, 2002).

Conclusions

For Planetree's principles of patient empowerment to be fully and meaningfully honored, CAM modalities simply must be made accessible to patients. If this occurs independently of conventional practice it will result in disconnected systems of care that have the potential for dangerous incompatibilities and regrettable gaps. Much is to be gained by overcoming the historical distinction between conventional and complementary care and instead thinking of care as properly involving all reasonable treatment options. The reasonableness of such options should be based on the thoughtful application of a hierarchy of evidence that pertains to safety, effectiveness, and alternatives as well as the beliefs and preferences of the patient.

Advances in integrative care have thus far occurred predominantly in the outpatient setting, and this trend will likely continue for some time. However, this approach to the incorporation of CAM modalities among treatment options is no less reasonable in the hospital setting. In the inpatient setting, the credentialing requirements for CAM practitioners would likely be more stringent and the scope of practice would be more limited. Even so, the options available to patients could be meaningfully enhanced. Progress toward more integrative inpatient care could very reasonably begin with the most accepted and evidence-based CAM modalities, including acupuncture, chiropractic, nutritional therapies, massage, and meditation, to name a few.

The challenges of achieving integrative medicine as the prevailing norm in modern health care are great. The reticence of the conventional medical establishment must be overcome. CAM practitioners must be prepared to find common ground, and common language, with their allopathic colleagues. All practitioners must embrace the importance and value of scientific evidence yet be willing to acknowledge its limits. Insurers will need to reimburse for those CAM modalities sanctioned by practitioners of integrative medicine before the public can realize any benefit. In support of this goal, cost-effective models of care will need to be developed.

Integrative care should continue its evolution in outpatient settings. As CAM and conventional modalities are successfully aligned for outpatients, these experiences should inform a gradual transformation of inpatient care, where the barriers are greater and the stakes are perhaps somewhat higher. Emphasis should be placed on CAM modalities that are best supported by evidence, for which credentialing and training are most stringent and for which the need is greatest, including naturopathic medicine, acupuncture, chiropractic, nutritional and herbal medicine, mind-body interventions, and therapeutic massage.

We are perhaps quite a long way from integrative care as the standard of practice in the United States. Yet the very trends that are reshaping modern health care—patient empowerment among them—may propel us in that direction. One can envision a day when the compatibility of treatment options with a patient's beliefs and values is a universal priority. One can envision a day when practitioners with varied training and expertise collaborate in a spirit of mutual respect. One can envision a day when evidence is universally valued and every practitioner acknowledges that patients should not be abandoned if their needs take them past evidence's leading edge.

It has been said that the single best way to predict the future is to create it. Perhaps, then, envisioning the advantages of integrative care is the first best step toward realizing them. Like conventional medicine, CAM includes therapies that are safe and effective, therapies that are the one but not the other, and therapies that are neither. Caution must therefore be exercised as CAM is integrated into established systems of inpatient and outpatient care. But the need to be cautious and thoughtful is no reason not to proceed. We should all aim for the day when there is no "alternative" or "conventional" care but rather just good options predicated on science, evidence, safety, effectiveness, and patient preferences and beliefs. When all of medicine is available to all patients, when responsibility and responsiveness are universally aligned, the center of care and the interests of the patient will truly coincide. Patient empowerment and the best achievable outcomes in health care will be realized when expert guidance to one continuous spectrum of treatment options is routinely available.

References

Angell, M., and Kassirer, J. "Alternative Medicine: The Risks of Untested and Unregulated Remedies." *New England Journal of Medicine*, 1998, 39, 839–841.

Astin, J., and others. "A Review of the Incorporation of Complementary and Alternative Medicine by Mainstream Physicians." *Archives of Internal Medicine*, 1998, 58, 2303–2310.

Beyerstein, B. "Alternative Medicine and Common Errors of Reasoning." *Academic Medicine*, 2001, 76, 230–237.

Dalen, J. "'Conventional' and 'Unconventional' Medicine." *Archives of Internal Medicine*, 1998, 158, 2179–2181.

Druss, B., and Rosenheck, R. "Association Between Use of Unconventional Therapies and Conventional Medical Services." *JAMA*, 1999, 282, 651–656.

Eisenberg, D., and others. "Unconventional Medicine in the United States." *New England Journal of Medicine*, 1993, 328, 246–252.

Eisenberg, D. M., and others, "Trends in Alternative Medicine Use in the United States, 1990–1997." *JAMA*, 1998, 280, 1569–1575.

Elder, N., Gillchrist, A., and Minz, R. "Use of Alternative Health Care by Family Practice Patients." *Archives of Family Medicine*, 1997, 6, 181–184.

Feldman, M. "Patients Who Seek Unorthodox Medical Treatment." *Minnesota Medicine*, 1990, 73, 19–25.

Harris, P., and Rees, R. "The Prevalence of Complementary and Alternative Medicine Use Among the General Population: A Systematic Review of the Literature." *Complementary Therapies in Medicine*, 2000, 8, 88–96.

Hemphill, L., and Kemp, J. "Implementing a Therapeutic Massage Program in a Tertiary and Ambulatory Care VA Setting: The Healing Power of Touch." *Nursing Clinics of North America*, 2000, 35, 489–497.

Katz, D. "Conventional Medical Care and Unconventional Therapies." *JAMA*, 1999, 281, 56.

Katz, D. *Clinical Epidemiology and Evidence-Based Medicine*. Thousand Oaks, Calif.: Sage, 2001.

Katz, D., and others. "Evidence Mapping: Introduction of Methods with Application to Complementary and Alternative Medicine Research." *Alternative Therapies in Health & Medicine*, 2002.

Kessler, R., and others. "Long-Term Trends in the Use of Complementary and Alternative Medical Therapies in the United States." *Annals of Internal Medicine*, 2001, 135, 262–268.

Marcus, D. "How Should Alternative Medicine Be Taught to Medical Students and Physicians?" *Academic Medicine*, 2001, *76*, 224–229.

McKee, J. "Holistic Health and the Critique of Western Medicine." *Social Science Medicine*, 1988, *26*, 775–784.

Mitchell, S. "Healing Without Doctors." *American Demographics*, 1993, *15*, 46–49.

Okvat, H., Oz, M., Ting, W., and Namerow, P. "Massage Therapy for Patients Undergoing Cardiac Catheterization." *Alternative Therapies in Health & Medicine*, 2002, *8*, 68–70, 72, 74–75.

Oz, M. "Emerging Role of Complementary Medicine in Valvular Surgery." *Advances in Cardiology*, 2002, *39*, 184–188.

Pelletier, K., Astin, J., and Haskell, W. "Current Trends in the Integration and Reimbursement of Complementary and Alternative Medicine by Managed Care Organizations (MCOs) and Insurance Providers: 1998 Update and Cohort Analysis." *American Journal of Health Promotion*, 1999, *14*, 125–133.

Pelletier, K., Marie, A., Krasner, M., and Haskell, W. "Current Trends in the Integration and Reimbursement of Complementary and Alternative Medicine by Managed Care, Insurance Carriers, and Hospital Providers." *American Journal of Health Promotion*, 1997, *12*, 112–122.

Perelson, G. "Alternative Medicine: What Role in Managed Care?" *Journal of Clinical Residency*, 1996, *5*, 32–38.

Rao, J., and others. "Use of Complementary Therapies for Arthritis Among Patients of Rheumatologists." *Annals of Internal Medicine*, 1999, *131*, 409–416.

Relman, A., and Weil, A. "Is Integrative Medicine the Medicine of the Future?" *Archives of Internal Medicine*, 1999, *159*, 2122–2126.

Sampson, W. "The Need for Educational Reform in Teaching About Alternative Therapies." *Academic Medicine*, 2001, *76*, 248–250.

U.S. Department of Health and Human Services. *Healthy People 2000: National Health and Promotion and Disease Prevention Objectives*. Washington, D.C.: U.S. Government Printing Office, 1991.

9

Healing Environments
Architecture and Design Conducive to Health

Bruce Arneill and Karrie Frasca-Beaulieu

Since its founding in 1978, Planetree has been dedicated to the transformation of the health care experience for patients and their families. The design and construction of health care facilities is only one of a number of critical components that can change a frightening institution into one that has a supportive and nurturing environment.

Some mistakenly believe that Planetree's goals can be achieved by focusing on a specific type of architecture or interior design, concluding that there is a Planetree "look" that includes the use of wood and other natural materials, indirect lighting, and homelike furnishings. But a beautiful health care unit is not necessarily one in which patients feel nurtured and supported. A patient who is frightened, lonely, and isolated from family and friends is not likely to notice the carefully decorated surroundings. It is only when the architecture and interior design works in concert with other Planetree components that the environment can help a caring staff help a patient feel less lonely and isolated.

One of Planetree's founding board members, Roslyn Lindheim, a professor of architecture at the University of California at Berkeley, designed the first Planetree model site. The thirteen-bed medical-surgical unit opened in 1985 at Pacific Presbyterian Medical Center in San Francisco. Lindheim's design concepts have become vital to the Planetree model, not simply for their architectural and aesthetic qualities but also because they have been shown to influence behaviors, interactions, and emotional responses.

Lindheim emphasized that the design of health care settings should

- Welcome the patient's family and friends

- Value human beings over technology

- Enable patients to fully participate as partners in their care

- Provide flexibility to personalize the care of each patient

- Encourage caregivers to be responsive to patients

- Foster a connection to nature and beauty

Throughout Planetree's history, these principles have been translated into a variety of health care settings, including emergency and intensive care departments, obstetrics, medical/surgical suites, and ambulatory care units, and they have been extended to entire facilities. They have been implemented in small rural hospitals, midsized community facilities, and large urban medical centers, always with the same goal: providing patients with an environment that is supportive of health and healing.

Planetree architecture is not confined to any particular style. It can be modern, eclectic, or contextual, and it can be applied to both new construction and renovations—to fit the predominant group and culture using it. More important, Planetree architecture does not celebrate the creativity of the architect over the users of the facility. What grew out of Lindheim's pioneering work was not a set of design rules to be duplicated again and again but rather a focus on the role of design as being integral to the patient's experience of health care. Planetree believes that design should not be the focus but rather a supporting element in the creation of a healing environment. Many Planetree hospitals have created patient-centered facilities with minimal renovation or new construction. Good design, however, can enhance Planetree concepts and support behavior consistent with patient-centered care.

Over the last two decades, the advent of the Planetree philosophy, as well as other societal changes, has sparked a revolution about the importance of health care facility design. In a major paradigm shift, sensitivity to people's feelings and their need for sensory input have entered the lexicon of facility planning and design. Competition among health care institutions, along with a concurrent evolution in hospitality design quality (in, for example, hotels and shopping malls), has created exciting opportunities for planning and designing facilities that are attractive and sensitive to the needs of both the patients and the staff.

Planetree Design

The holistic approach to healing espoused by Planetree moves beyond regarding the human body as a machine and the hospital as a repair shop. In the conventional model, the patient is a body that the practitioner is going to *work on*. According to Planetree, the patient is a whole person (body/mind/spirit) whom the practitioner is going to *work with*. To support this model, the hospital or health care delivery environment should be designed using the following principles.

Stress Reduction

In 1991, in a careful, well-controlled experiment at Carnegie Mellon University, researchers examined the direct link between stress and illness. The landmark study, published in the *New England Journal of Medicine*, provided the first scientific demonstration that stress can increase the risk of infection (Falk and Woods, 1973). Just as stress can influence the onset of illness and opportunistic diseases, research also suggests that stress-reducing environments can have an effect on healing. Studies have linked poor facility design to elevated blood pressure, anxiety, delirium, nausea, the increased need for medication, and longer hospital stays following surgery (Ulrich, 1992; Malkin, 1992; Maslow and Mintz, 1965; Knapp and others, 1993).

First Impressions Set by the Parking and Lobby Experience

Simply driving to a health facility can build fear and anxiety, so a patient's initial impression may depend on something as basic as a good set of directions. Since most health care centers have several entrances, including emergency, main lobby, ambulatory services, birthing centers, and other support services, access to the desired destination should be clear and easily comprehensible.

Parking can also be a major frustration for health facility users, particularly when combined with the anxieties and infirmities of a health- or age-related problem. Immediate, well-marked parking, combined with a covered drop-off, helps ensure a positive impression and minimizes frustration. Where parking spaces are limited, a valet parking system should be considered.

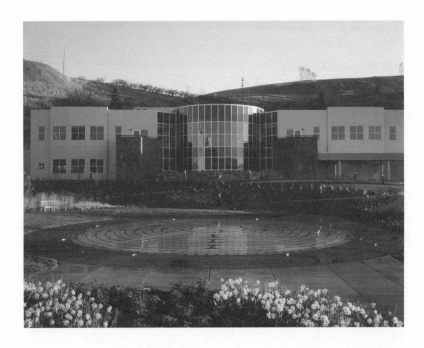

The first image of the facility occurs at the site's entrance, and the first contact is with those assisting parking and direction finding. These initial "ten-second" contacts can set the tone for all future facility impressions. Entry, parking, wayfinding, and signage are key aspects of a well-designed site; but it is important to remember that these elements support and enhance a friendly, helping staff.

Other exterior characteristics include attractive and well-maintained landscaping and site lighting. Restful, calming music, even in parking and entry areas, helps set the initial ambience. Approaching a Planetree facility should not be very different from approaching a fine hotel or a beautiful spa, known for its superior service and amenities.

Given the stresses that many patients and families are under, entering a Planetree facility should be as welcoming and non-threatening as possible. The entrance should be human-scaled and visibly defined by a pleasant covered entry that protects patients and visitors from inclement weather. Music should be heard in

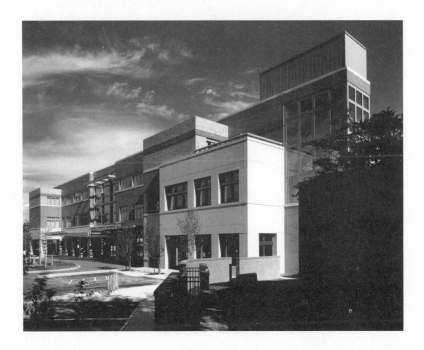

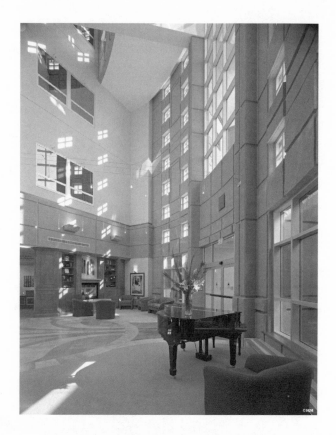

reception areas, creating a calming, soothing environment and muffling random noise. Atriums have become a common feature in hospital design, but a comforting, intimate space with a simple concierge desk also creates an appropriate ambience in a Planetree facility. A personal interaction with the reception staff can be especially critical in establishing the welcoming, service-oriented environment.

The lobby of a Planetree facility must provide access to clear, comprehensible circulation pathways. At some sites, the health resource center, which serves as a communal library and meeting place for patients, family, community groups, and schools, is centrally located off the lobby. Access to this key public function is ide-

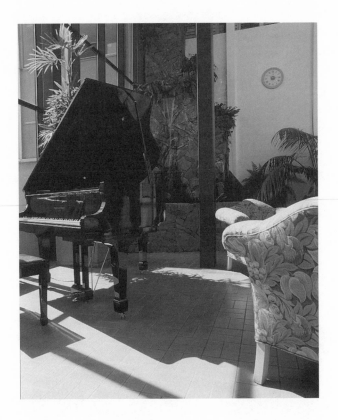

ally convenient from the main entrance, perhaps even preempting the typical priority of the hospital gift shop.

Getting Around the Facility

Many times, wayfinding in a health care facility is an afterthought and consists only of signage. Wayfinding in a Planetree facility should be a combination of signage, architectural elements, lighting, color, artwork, and furniture. Public spaces can be clearly differentiated from private spaces with glass doors and sidelights, whereas rooms that are off-limits to the public can have painted doors that blend into the corridors.

Accent lighting, such as pendants and sconces, as well as ceiling design, can also play an important role in wayfinding by highlighting

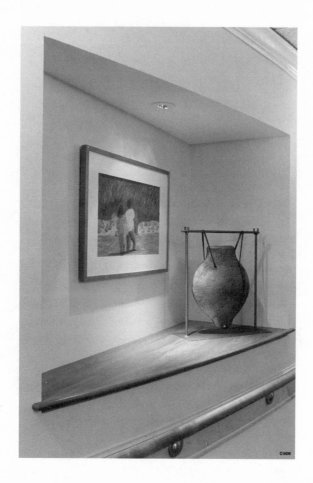

key destinations, such as elevator lobbies, nursing stations, and intersections. A striking piece of furniture or artwork can be a help-ful landmark. Using a combination of these elements creates unmis-takable points of reference that help people navigate. The faster patients are oriented to their environment and able to find their destination, the greater their sense of control and reduction of stress.

Access to Nature

Clinical research suggests that viewing nature scenes can reduce blood pressure and muscle tension. Moreover, it is well known that people need exposure to daylight for their physiological and psychological well-being. This is particularly true for people whose illness requires a prolonged stay indoors. In fact, research on intensive care units has shown that rooms without windows aggravate the deleterious effects of environmental stimulation caused by unvarying lighting and the repetitive sounds of respirators and other equipment. But even if this research were inconclusive, each of us knows, firsthand, the soothing effects of a cool breeze, summer sunset, or gently falling rain (Marberry, 1997; Ulrich, 1992).

The waiting area for ambulatory surgery and endoscopy at Lakeland Hospital, in Niles, Michigan, is designed to focus the attention of patients and families toward the calming and peaceful view provided by the natural setting of the St. Joseph River. Through a saw toothed, angled plan, patients and their families are able to settle into a semi-private portion of the waiting room and look through wide, engaging windows onto nature as they mentally prepare for their procedure. This view, natural light, quiet acoustics, and calming music all contribute to an environment where the patient can become less anxious.

Through the use of courtyards, rooftop gardens, and terraces, designers are beginning to use the power of nature indoors, helping patients relax their minds, bodies, and spirits. In the ICU at Griffin Hospital in Derby, Connecticut, the visitor corridor has glass block windows, enabling patients to maintain their privacy but also taking advantage of natural light.

Nurturing and Supportive Environments

In a hospital setting, it is extremely important for patients to feel connected with the staff if they are to feel less anxious and more supported in their health care experience. Nevertheless, it is not unusual to see large nursing stations on a typical patient unit, set apart from patients by half-walls or glass partitions. These elements clearly send a message that staff members are distancing themselves from patients or that they are busy and inaccessible.

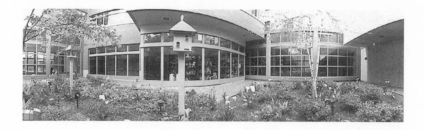

The Planetree philosophy, on the other hand, encourages patients and families to be involved with the staff and participating in the healing process. For example, at several Planetree facilities, there are small, open nursing stations outside each cluster of four to six rooms, with the main nursing station completely open to patients. In fact, these nursing stations are simply tables and chairs in the center of the space. This arrangement suggests that healing is not something that happens *to* patients, it is something that happens *with them*. Staff members are not only accessible; they are also there to collaborate and confer with each patient about health and healing.

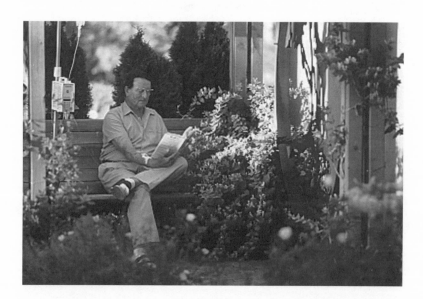

Comfort Zones

The reception and lounge areas of each major hospital department need to maintain the Planetree ambiance established at the facility's main entrance. These reception areas serve as zones for quiet relaxation, providing comfort for both patients and family members. It is important to note, however, that the definition of comfort can vary, depending on the service or department.

Comfort can be achieved by familiarity and expectations. The main reception area for Lakeland's Niles campus is located in the heart of the intersection of four clinical wings directly in view from the main entry. Patients and families walk by the entry garden and are greeted by a receptionist who is expecting them and directs them to the appropriate outpatient or inpatient clinical area. Scattered seating areas around the reception desk provide a variety of waiting options yet keeps one visually linked to the main reception. The resource center is directly adjacent so patients and families have the option of doing research using video or written materials as they wait for their appointment or a family member.

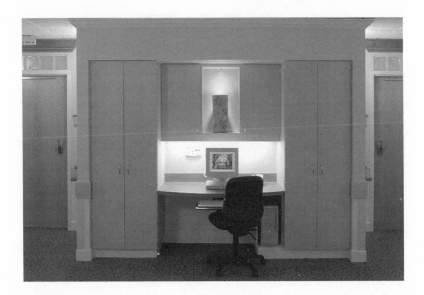

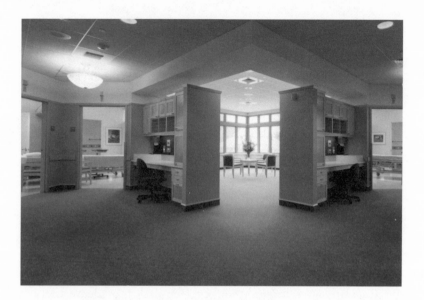

• In ambulatory care and outpatient services, comfort includes confidence that appointments will stay on schedule and that waiting times will be short. Lounge spaces should not have a blaring TV and a crowded seating area. Attractive interior design elements can include natural light, artwork, and water features, such as fountains or tropical fish tanks. At the emergency department of Bergan Mercy Medical Center in Omaha, Nebraska, a centrally located fountain produces white sound to increase confidentiality between the reception desk and the waiting area.

• A birthing center should comfort new mothers, fathers, and extended family members. The birthing center ambiance should extend from reception, through clear wayfinding, to comfortable homelike bedrooms. Design considerations should include live-in spaces for baby and father and special menus for "nonhospital" meals. Some facilities provide Jacuzzis.

The acute care units have similar lounge and reception requirements. Seating need not be extensive, but it should have a residen-

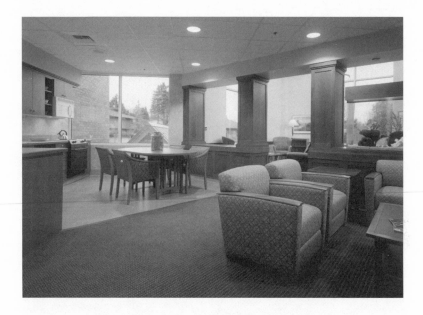

tial feeling. Because corridors serve a range of functions, the use of cul-de-sacs and modules for bedroom clusters can help reduce their length and minimize their institutional quality. Intensive care units can benefit from *clutter corridors*—that is, service spaces that contain all the medical equipment that can congest conventional corridors. Acute care bedrooms should be as residential as possible, with comfortable seating as well as convertible bed/couches for family members. Acute care floors should offer small lounge areas for respite and quiet time for family members. Since Planetree emphasizes family participation in the healing process, there is a need for private discussion and interaction spaces.

Education and Personal Growth

In the Planetree approach, patients are encouraged to become active participants in their own healing process. Patients are not expected to comply with instructions passively, as wellness is considered an educational process. Professional staff members enlist patients as partners in a healing program that encompasses mind,

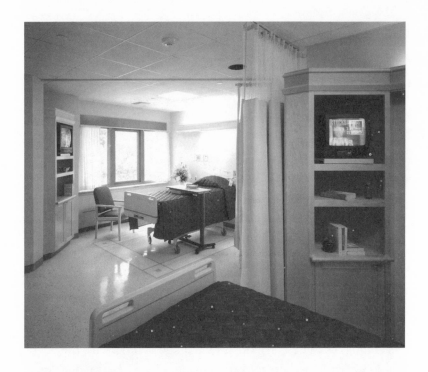

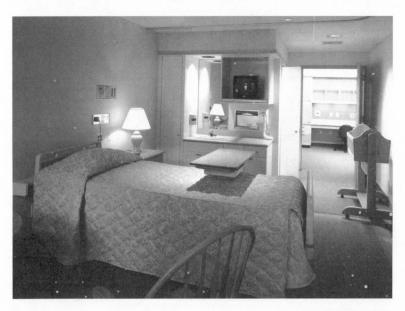

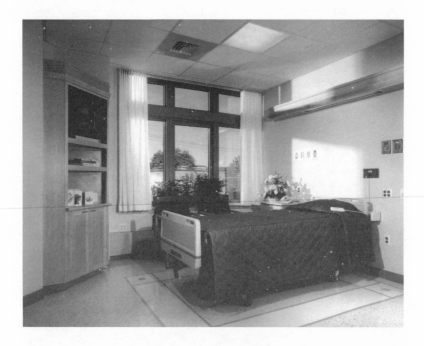

body, and spirit. Healing comes not only from modern technology, diagnosis, pharmaceuticals, and procedures; it also flows from an environment that encourages personal growth and development, positive attitudes, emotional well-being, healthy human relationships, community, spirituality, and joy.

In a Planetree environment, patients are urged to read their own charts and understand their diagnoses, treatment options, and medications, as well as preventive practices for wellness. Open discussions with the staff are encouraged by the configuration of nursing stations, and health education is fostered by the presence of health resources centers or unit libraries. At Griffin Hospital, a two-story glass-enclosed resource center is the main focal point of the hospital, containing a library for each floor, with an area for viewing educational videotapes as well as an area for computers with Internet access. Classroom spaces and audiovisual rooms were created for

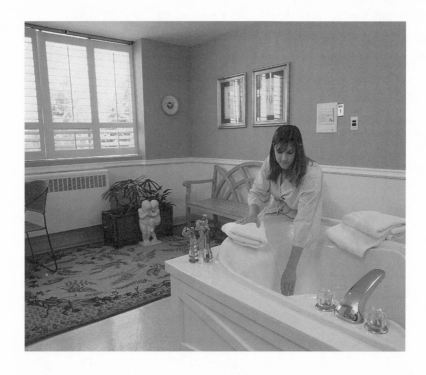

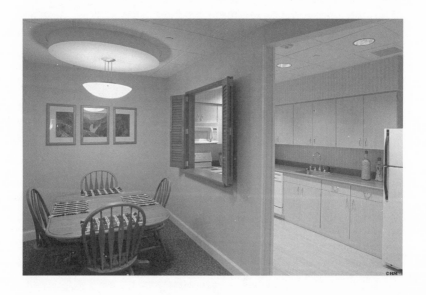

wellness programs, including those for nutrition and exercise, as well as stress-reduction classes.

Family Participation

In the Planetree philosophy is the belief that family, friends, and the community play a vital role in the healing process and that wellness is generated by positive human relationships, community spirit, and emotional well-being. Research has indicated that strong social support can reduce stress and accelerate healing. It is therefore essential for designers of Planetree facilities to accommodate patients and their loved ones.

Comfortable overnight accommodations, visitor areas, and lounge/activity rooms help patients feel close to their family and friends. The family rooms and kitchens should be located close to patient rooms and should be comfortably furnished. The main

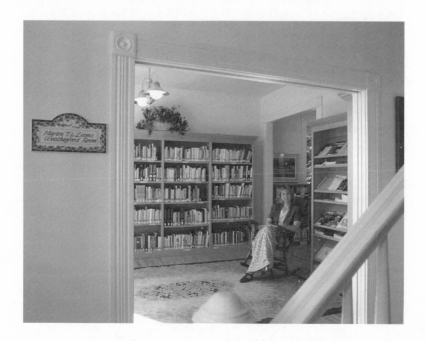

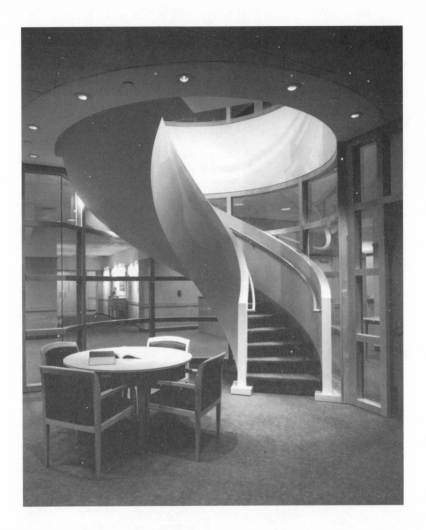

furniture groups (sofas and lounge chairs) should be arranged to foster social interaction, and other seating can be arranged for intimate conversations. The family rooms should have areas to view
television as well as tables and chairs for reading.

ICUs can be high-energy work environments that quickly create stress in both patients and family members. The ICU design of
Griffin Hospital separates the high-tech staff area from the visitor
area by adding a separate entrance to each patient room through a

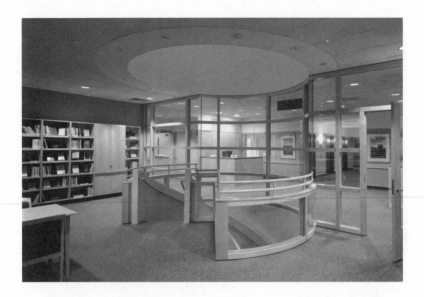

corridor along the perimeter of the unit. In this way, family members can remain close to patients without undue stress or disrupting the medical staff. Along this corridor are lounges, small kitchenettes, bathrooms, and terraces for family members and friends to use while visiting their loved ones.

Patients typically feel that they have limited control over what and how they eat while in the hospital. In a Planetree facility, small residential-type kitchens can be located on each unit so that patients and families have the option of preparing their own meals or snacks. Even when patients' diets are restricted by doctor's orders, these kitchens can be used to teach sound nutrition and healthy food preparation techniques. Family members are encouraged to participate, so that once patients leave the facility, they continue their lifestyle changes.

Engaging the Senses

The Planetree philosophy celebrates the importance of the five senses. This attention to sensory input should begin at the edge of the building site and seamlessly continue into the facility itself. In

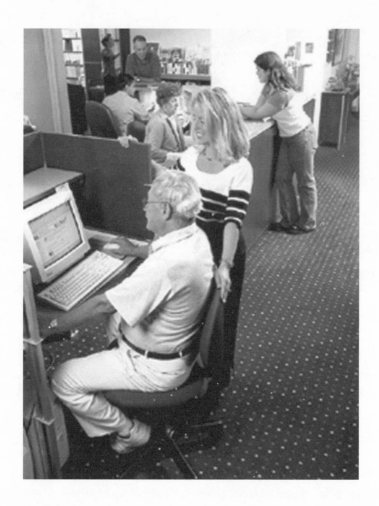

progressing from parking to entry to lobby and then entering into the health facility, what one sees, hears, smells, touches, and tastes is vital to a holistic, thoughtful, patient-centered environment.

Sound

Reducing the amount of noise is an important factor to be considered in the creation of a healing environment. Sound can be negative if it is perceived as noise and cannot be controlled; in fact, noise is one of the most significantly detrimental environmental factors known to cause physiological changes in the body and affect healing. From the reverberation of intercoms to the beeping of cardiac machines, hospi-

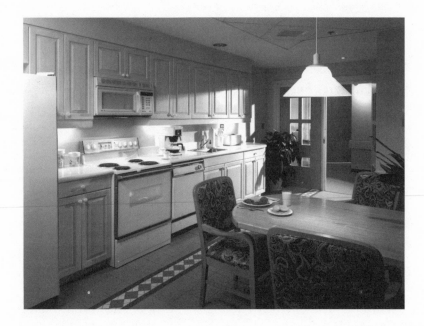

tal sounds can be discomforting and disturbing for patients who have
to listen to them. Designers may not be able to eliminate stress-induc-
ing noises, but they can certainly attempt to reduce them. Carpeting is
a good solution in corridors, lessening the impact of footsteps, rolling
equipment, and random conversations. Locating utility rooms and
equipment storage areas away from patient rooms can also help eliminate disturbing sounds. Internal corridors can be located between utility and storage rooms so that nursing and maintenance personnel will
not disturb patients. Such private corridors, removed from patients
and visitors, reduce the noise pollution typically associated with the
hustle and bustle of hospital operations (Malkin, 1992).

Music can be an integral part of the healing process, providing
a positive distraction to patients' perception of noise. As patients
tune into the music, they can more easily tune out annoying sounds.
From the moment patients and visitors open their car doors in the
hospital parking lot, they should be invited into the facility with
lyrical gestures. They can be greeted by a player piano in the lobby
or hear strolling musicians on patient units.

Texture

The use of different textures is also important to minimizing the institutional feel of a hospital. Our homes are filled with a variety of rich textures, and the presence of different tactile elements can remind patients of home. To establish a residential feel, designers can use sculpture, upholstery with tactile patterns, and textured vinyl wall covering, as well as wood furnishings and cabinetry, throughout a health care facility.

Lighting

Natural light connects interior spaces with the world outside, and one key to a pleasant interior is to provide as much natural light as possible. In a health care facility, it is especially important to include control systems for natural light that respond to changing conditions. The intensity and high contrast of uncontrolled natural light can actually impair vision, especially in older people. The use of draperies and blinds are an essential feature in patient rooms to foster patients' sense of control over their environment. These window coverings not only adjust the amount of light that enters the room, they also allow patients to establish a sense of privacy.

Improper lighting can be a major source of psychological and physical stress on patients. Excessively bright or glaring lights can cause headaches and nausea, whereas lack of lighting has been known to cause fatigue and depression. Proper lighting should accommodate the requirements of the space, but lights should be alterable by patients so as not to limit their sense of control. Using a variety of lights and lighting levels can accommodate the clinical tasks at hand while providing flexibility, control, and comfort. For example, in patient rooms it may be necessary to have bright overhead examination lights available, but patients should be able to shut them off when they are not in use. General lighting should also be controllable to allow patients to choose the ambiance they desire. It is also recommended that patient reading lamps be made available on each bedside table.

It is equally important for visitor areas to have appropriate lighting. Typically, two- by four-foot fluorescent fixture lights are used in these areas, creating a glaring environment not conducive to relaxation. By using a combination of different types of lighting, such as recessed fluorescent downlighting for general illumination, accent wallwashers to highlight artwork, and floor and table lamps for reading, designers can create a residential atmosphere that feels more comfortable, supportive, and nurturing.

Color

It is difficult to separate color from lighting because the appearance of color depends on levels of illumination and the spectral distribution of the light source. Designers must examine a variety of interrelated factors concerning color in order to create spaces that are warm, caring, friendly, supportive, and technically proficient. Among important color questions to ask are:

- Do the colors reduce the institutional look?

- Do they reinforce the philosophy of the hospital?

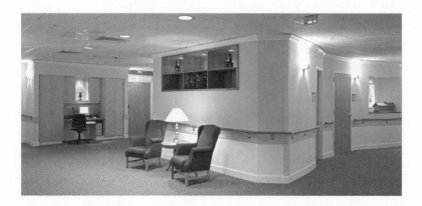

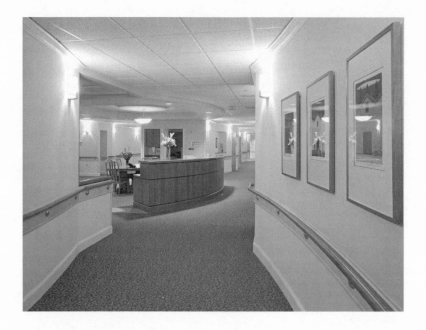

- Do they support wayfinding?

- Do they support the function of the space by enhancing visual acuity and the accuracy of examinations or diagnoses?

- Do they reduce or induce stress?

- Are they sensitive to different populations using the space (such as the elderly, children, minorities, or members of different cultures and religions) as well as to their illnesses/disorders?

- Do they create a visually interesting, aesthetically pleasing, and stimulating environment?

- Do they take into consideration the geographical location of the hospital and the building's orientation to the sun?

There are no rules about specific color selections for a hospital, but there has been an abundance of research on the psychological, biological, and physiological effects of color. This should be considered, but it is ultimately the designer's interpretation of this information as well as his or her taste and talent that makes an environment successful.

Smell and Taste

One of the more unusual aspects of many Planetree facilities is a pleasant, small kitchen on the nursing unit or in the ambulatory care and maternity center. Staff members and volunteers make a point of providing patients and visitors with coffee, tea, and perhaps even a fresh chocolate chip cookie. The aroma of baked goods from volunteer bakers is not only pleasant, but it can also help mask "institutional" odors typically experienced in health care facilities.

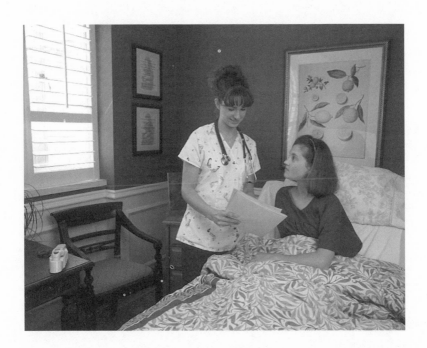

The sense of taste can also be served by offering bowls of healthy candies and snacks in the lobby and reception areas, as well as in snack kitchens and the main dining area.

Sacred Space

Designing sacred space in a health care facility is much more than providing an ecumenical chapel, strategically located and easily accessible. Being in a space that promotes serenity and peace can produce a spiritual infusion much like a blood transfusion, and areas of sanctuary and refuge for family, staff members, and patients are extremely important in a Planetree facility. Designers should make a priority of providing peaceful spaces for meditation, reflection, and self-examination, such as courtyards and terraces with flower gardens, benches, and labyrinths. Throughout the facility, such amenities as fish tanks and fountains should be considered, to help patients reestablish a sense of harmony at a time when they need it most.

The concept of sacred space also extends to enabling a patient to transform an area of his or her room into a personalized place that conveys a sense of harmony and belongingness. For example, special shelves and bulletin boards in the patient's room enable the patient to display flowers, cards, and gifts and view them from his or her bed. Ideally, the entire hospital should create a sense of sacred space.

Conclusion

Since 1978, Planetree has been helping health care facilities transform themselves from high-tech, sterile, treatment-oriented institutions to warm, comfortable, nurturing, people-centered healing environments. Their approach has forced us to reconsider the elements of good design, recognizing the vital link between the physical space and the healing process. In addition to the complex interrelation of mind, body, and spirit, it has helped us appreciate the profundity of our connection with nature and with others.

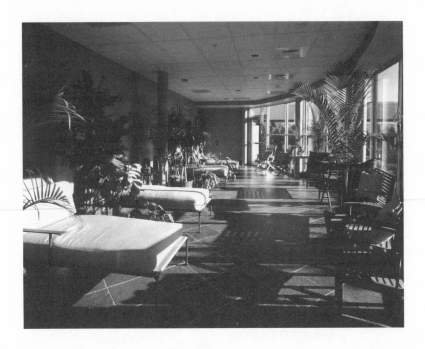

As we continue into the twenty-first century, we must broaden our understanding of these connections and integrate rapidly changing technologies into the Planetree vision of truly holistic centers of healing. Thoughtful facility design not only actualizes a philosophy of care, it can also ensure that our health care institutions are efficient, orderly, and functional—and at the same time stress-reducing, supportive, user-friendly, comfortable, and healing. Design that is truly sensitive to the Planetree concept will encourage behavior changes, help refocus staff energies, and, most important, empower patients and families to realize their full healing potential.

References

Falk and Woods. "Effects of Noise in Recovery Rooms." *New England Journal of Medicine*, 1973, *189*(15), 774–481.

Knapp, P. H., and others. "Moods, Emotions Impact Immunity, Mental Medicine Update." *The Mind/Body Health Newsletter*, Spring 1993, Vol. II, p. 1.

Malkin, J. *Hospital Interior Architecture: Creating Healing Environments for Special Patient Populations*. New York: Van Nostrand Reinhold, 1992.

Marberry, S. (ed.). *Healthcare Design*. New York: Wiley, 1997.

Maslow, A., and Mintz, N. C. "Effect of Aesthetics on Perception." *Journal of Psychology*, 1965, *41*, 247–254.

Ulrich, R. S. "How Design Impacts Wellness." *Healthcare Forum Journal*, Sep./Oct. 1992, p. 24.

Part Two

Future Directions for
Patient-Centered Care

10

Building the Business Case
for Patient-Centered Care

Patrick A. Charmel

Since its inception as a demonstration project serving as a model of patient-centered care delivery, the founders of the Planetree model and their successors have been continually challenged to demonstrate its efficacy and value. Many of Planetree's early adopters found the model's underlying philosophy compelling. They were willing to adopt the model's programmatic elements based on an inherent belief that the delivery of personalized, compassionate care in a healing environment was "the right thing to do." However, many decision makers have subjected the Planetree approach to greater scrutiny. They have demanded documentation of the tangible benefits to be derived from adoption of the model. In particular, skeptics have asked for data substantiating a fair return on the investment of time, energy (both physical and emotional), and money necessary to implement Planetree and achieve its benefits. Until now, the Planetree model's value proposition has not been clearly articulated. Failure to proffer a strong business case for the Planetree model has impeded its widespread adoption. However, data do indeed exist that substantiate the business benefits of patient-centered care. A review of the evolution of the Planetree model and a description of the rigor to which it was subjected as a condition of its development are helpful in establishing a foundation from which to build a credible business case.

Demonstrating Planetree's Effectiveness

The Planetree Model Hospital Unit was established in 1985 at the then 272-bed Pacific Presbyterian Medical Center (PPMC) in San Francisco, with funding from The San Francisco Foundation and The Kaiser Family Foundation, to demonstrate the benefits of patient-centered care and to serve as a model for hospital and health care providers throughout the country. The founders of Planetree and the foundations that funded its development recognized that to gain acceptance in an industry dominated by the scientific method, patient-centered care would have to demonstrate its superiority to traditional care, using a methodology that would withstand scientific scrutiny.

Researchers from the University of Washington School of Public Health were commissioned to conduct a randomized controlled trial to compare the patient outcomes on the Planetree Model Hospital Unit with those on PPMC's other medical-surgical units. The University of Washington study is believed to be the first comprehensive evaluation of patient outcomes on a patient-centered unit, compared with a traditional unit, ever conducted. Outcome indicators chosen by the researchers included patient satisfaction, patient education and involvement in the care process, patient health behavior and compliance, health status and hospital resource consumption (defined as length of stay), and hospital charges generated (Martin and others, 1998).

Patients were enrolled in the study for a period lasting more than three years, from late 1986 to early 1990. A total of 760 patients participated, 315 of whom were cared for on the Planetree unit, with 445 being cared for on other medical-surgical units. Study subjects underwent a thorough twenty-minute interview upon admission and completed written questionnaires one week, three months, and six months after discharge. In addition, hospital bills were analyzed to quantify resource consumption during the initial hospital admission and subsequent hospital stays. Consumption of nonacute care services, such as home care, emergency room care, and ambulatory care in the year following enrollment in the study were also quantified.

The findings indicated that patients had significantly higher overall satisfaction on the Planetree Unit than on the other units studied, they had greater opportunity to see family and friends, they were more satisfied with their nursing care and the unit's architecture and environment, they learned more about their illness and self-care, and they were included more often in the care process. In addition, Planetree patients were more satisfied with the health education they received while hospitalized. Theses findings left no doubt that the model of care delivery was effective. However, for the remaining performance indicators studied, the Planetree unit failed to demonstrate an advantage.

Study participants cared for on the Planetree unit experienced essentially the same length of stay as patients on the other units. Charges generated, a proxy for hospital resources consumed, were also similar. Although study findings indicated that Planetree unit patients learned more about their illness and self-care requirements, that knowledge did not translate into improved health status or decreased use of inpatient hospital services and ambulatory services in the year following study enrollment. It is safe to say that given the hospital industry's relentless pursuit of operating cost reduction, had the study found that engaging patients in the care process offered lasting benefits in terms of reduced use of health services, there would have been few obstacles to widespread adoption of the model. Although clear patient benefits have been demonstrated, the failure to show a clear cost advantage through improved operating efficiency necessitates the identification of other ways by which the model can improve its economic viability.

The Industry Shifts Its Focus

Faced with growing federal budget deficits and the prospect that the demands of an aging baby boom generation might bankrupt the Medicare program, Congress passed the Balanced Budget Amendment

(BBA) in 1997, in hopes of cutting the rate of Medicare expense growth in half. The BBA exceeded the expectation of Congress, in that in the years immediately following its adoption, real Medicare expense growth declined for the first time since the program's inception. The dramatic reduction in Medicare spending was achieved primarily through reductions in payments to hospitals and physicians. The resulting loss of revenue reduced the profitability of all hospitals. More than a third of the nation's hospitals with thin operating margins saw their profitability disappear altogether. In reaction, hospitals aggressively cut their operating costs through efficiency enhancement and productivity improvement.

Efficiency of care delivery was enhanced primarily through length-of-stay reduction. Length-of-stay reduction was achieved by standardizing the care of patients with a similar diagnosis to eliminate, to the extent possible, variability among physicians. Practice guidelines, also called care pathways, were the principle tool used to standardize care.

Reduction in the average length of stay and the associated reduction in the average daily census of the typical U.S. hospital facilitated labor cost savings through staff reductions. The need to compensate for lost Medicare revenue drove many hospitals to eliminate staff members to a greater degree than was justified by reduction in workload resulting from shorter average length of stay. To the dismay of hospital executives, productivity improvement—that is, producing more work with less staff—was insufficient to restore profitability or enhance operating margins. It soon became apparent that economic viability could only be assured by a strategy that combined cost reduction with revenue enhancement.

The hospital industry's shift of emphasis to revenue enhancement and business growth corresponded with the first appearances of the health care consumer movement. It has been said that health care consumerism will "alter how health care organizations operate, how they compete and, perhaps, why they exist" (Ernst & Young LLP, 1998) A growing appreciation that success through revenue enhancement and business growth cannot be achieved without responding to the forces of health care consumerism has motivated hospital leaders to become more customer focused. It may be that the Planetree model's greatest value is that it was designed from the health care consumers' perspective, and therefore it is most effective in responding to the health care consumer movement.

Health Care Consumerism

Health care consumerism is the collective expression of consumer demand for more responsive care and service by a growing mass of educated and empowered consumers (Ernst & Young LLP, 1998; KPMG Peat Marwick LLP, 1998). Health care consumerism is being driven by changes in society, improved access to information, and changes in the financing of health care. As levels of affluence have risen, consumers who are working more hours and have less free time have begun to demand improved service and convenience. The Internet has given consumers access to health care information and decision-making tools that enable them to play a more active role in their own health care. Finally, consumers have been given a choice of health insurance plans by government and private employers, but they are being asked to pay a larger share of the cost of their own health care. As consumers pay out of pocket for more of their care, they have begun to seek value in their health care purchases, as they do in other major purchases that they make. In general, consumers are willing to pay more for a product or service of higher perceived quality. Currently, in health care, the patient equates customer service with quality. Therefore, valued providers are those that deliver an exceptional patient experience.

The findings of the University of Washington study, mentioned earlier, and the patient satisfaction ratings in Planetree Alliance hospitals throughout the United States document the success of the Planetree model in meeting patient demand for more responsive care and service. A study of the patient satisfaction rates of twelve

Planetree hospitals—both one year prior to and two years following implementation of the model—indicated an average improvement rate across all hospitals studied of three or more percentage points in "overall satisfaction," "likeliness to recommend," and "willingness to return" (Iacono, 2002). The dramatic impact of the Planetree model on patient satisfaction is best depicted by the following chart, which displays the improvement in the rating of "overall satisfaction" by patients at Griffin Hospital, a 160-bed community teaching hospital and Planetree flagship hospital, since the adoption of the Planetree model.

Product Differentiation

Those hospitals that believe sustainable growth can come from offering services that exceed health care consumer expectations have chosen to differentiate themselves from hospitals in their market, based on their level of responsiveness to these expectations. In essence, they are building a brand identity around a patient-centered approach to care. That identity begins with a brand promise. The

Griffin Hospital Patient Satisfaction

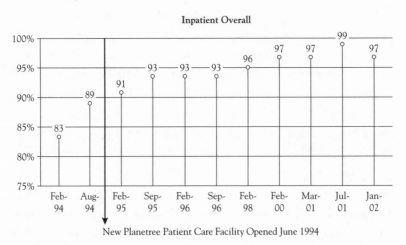

Inpatient Overall

New Planetree Patient Care Facility Opened June 1994

brand promise has three elements: product quality, reputation, and service. Brand identity and customer loyalty to a brand occur over a long period of time, often measured in years. This means that an organization must make a long-term commitment to the elements of the brand promise (Pine and Gilmore, 1999; Baker, 1998).

Hospitals that adopt the Planetree model have a strong belief in the model's underlying philosophy, which helps them maintain their commitment and overcome obstacles to model implementation. The cultural transformation that occurs in hospitals that embrace the philosophy occurs over a period of three to five years. Planetree Alliance members often refer to Planetree model implementation as a journey rather than a destination. Knowing that implementation is a long-term commitment prevents hospitals from adopting Planetree as a "quick fix" strategy. The Planetree model, with its focus on service quality and sustainability and its ability to define an organization and build its reputation, may be the ideal branding strategy in the era of health care consumerism.

Growing Public Accountability

Hospitals have to deal not only with growing health care consumerism but also with increasing public concern over medical errors and other adverse events. These issues have been reported by the Institute of Medicine in its widely circulated report "To Err is Human," as well as in various published investigative reports (Kohn, Corrigan, and Donaldson, 2000). This publicity has resulted in a cry for greater public accountability by the nation's hospitals. State legislators and regulators have responded by passing legislation or adopting regulations that require hospitals to submit clinical and customer service quality data. These data are to be incorporated into a comparative report of hospital performance, for release to the general public. Currently, eighteen states publish hospital report cards. Performance indicators include patient satisfaction rates, morbidity and mortality rates, medical error rates, and human resource data, such as nurse staffing ratios, vacancy rates, and turnover rates. The adoption of hospital report cards by the states, and the prospect that the federal government through the Medicare program may follow suit, pushes service enhancement beyond a differentiation strategy to an imperative necessary to ensure continued operation.

Failure to meet consumer expectations for customer service and clinical quality has serious implications beyond harm to the image and reputation of a hospital and loss of patient loyalty. With increasing frequency, patients with untoward outcomes are taking legal action against their caregivers. The settlements and jury awards in such cases are growing. A combination of factors, not the least of which is the number and size of medical malpractice payouts, has prompted insurers to dramatically increase their malpractice premiums or to exit the malpractice insurance marketplace altogether. This is leaving little competition between remaining companies and creating an environment for even greater premium increases down the road. The "medical malpractice crisis," as it has been called, has resulted in premium increases in 2002 that range from 50 to 300 percent. For many hospitals, this equates to millions of dollars in increased operating cost. The cost increases have been devastating to most hospitals, and stabilization of hospital rates is not expected in the near future.

Insurance underwriters base a hospital's malpractice insurance premium on a combination of industry experience and a hospital's individual claims history. Research shows that 1 percent of hospital patients nationwide are harmed in some way, but only 3 percent of those who are harmed file a lawsuit. Those who do sue do so because of one of four types of communication problems: deserting the patient, devaluing the patient's views, delivering information poorly, and failing to understand the patient's perspective (Kavalier and Spiegel, 1997).

The Planetree model's emphasis on improved caregiver-patient communication, patient and family involvement in the care process, and focus on the patient's perspective has the potential to

All Departments (By Policy Years 1994–2001 [9 mos.])
Adjusted Discharges vs. Number of Claims

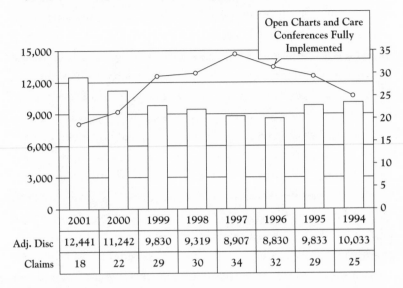

	2001	2000	1999	1998	1997	1996	1995	1994
Adj. Disc	12,441	11,242	9,830	9,319	8,907	8,830	9,833	10,033
Claims	18	22	29	30	34	32	29	25

reduce malpractice claims and associated operating cost increases. Although no study has been conducted to date on the impact of the Planetree model on malpractice claims, one hospital has reported compelling results. The chart above displays a dramatic reduction in malpractice claims in the years since adoption of the Planetree model, despite a large increase in patient care activity.

The Health Care Workforce Shortage

Health care consumerism is not the only force with which health care organizations have to contend. A growing health care workforce shortage is making it increasingly difficult to staff hospitals, which is jeopardizing patient safety and causing upward pressure on wages. The American Hospital Association Commission on Workforce report released in April 2002 states that, nationwide, the average vacancy rate for nurses, radiology technologists, and pharmacists is greater than 10 percent. One in seven hospitals has vacancy rates of 20 percent or more. Hospitals with high vacancy rates are forced to use temporary labor and pay a premium of more than double their standard rate for the privilege. Many of those who have chosen to avoid or who cannot afford to use agency staffing have been forced to turn away patients because of reduced capacity. Given the high fixed costs of operating a hospital, the resulting loss of revenue has been devastating.

Hospitals where employees are more satisfied and feel a sense of pride in their work have lower employee turnover and lower vacancy rates. The link between employee satisfaction and patient satisfaction has been well documented (Press Ganey Associates, 1999). The Press Ganey study found that open communication, pride in work, and exceptional management practices are more relevant to employee satisfaction than wages, benefits, and the work environment. The level of pride felt was the highest predictor of overall employee satisfaction. The fact that the Planetree philosophy resonates with so many caregivers, in that it focuses the attention and resources of the hospital on the needs of the patient, contributes to a strong sense of employee pride and high employee satisfaction in Planetree affiliate hospitals. As a result, vacancy rates at many Planetree sites are much lower than industry averages. New Jersey's Hackensack University Medical Center has a nurse vacancy rate under 10 percent, Warren Memorial Hospital in Front Royal, Virginia, has a nurse vacancy rate under 5 percent, and the same can be said for Mid-Columbia Medical Center in The Dalles, Oregon. Finally, Griffin Hospital in Derby, Connecticut, is one of only four hospitals to appear on the *Fortune Magazine* 2003 list entitled "The 100 Best Companies to Work for in America." It is the only hospital to appear on the list four years in a row. The *Fortune* designation is largely based on the results of a survey of employee pride and satisfaction, turnover, and vacancy rates.

The cost of employee turnover to a hospital has been quantified by the Health Care Advisory Board in Washington, D.C. It is estimated that the loss of one registered nurse costs a hospital an average of $29,265, which includes recruitment, new hire training, and the replacement labor cost and does not include the cost of lost revenue if capacity is diminished. To avoid the burdensome cost of turnover, hospitals must create an organization that is responsive to the needs of patients and their caregivers.

In Conclusion: A Strong Business Case

It has taken approximately two decades and the experience of more than sixty affiliates for the economic benefits of the Planetree model to become clear. Ironically, it may have been the hospital industry's failure to embrace a patient-centered approach that made the need for Planetree and similar models so apparent when the hospital-operating environment became hostile. The industry's commitment to the status quo and its unwillingness to embrace the patient and the patient's family members as partners in the care and healing process resulted in indifferent and unresponsive care, alienated and dissatisfied health care consumers, and disenchanted and unfulfilled providers. The cost to hospitals has been enormous, as described earlier.

The shift of focus and the investment of time, attention, and resources necessary to adopt and implement the Planetree model, while not insignificant, are dwarfed by the economic benefit of an improved competitive position in the marketplace. This is achieved through product differentiation, the development of brand loyalty, improved liability claims experience, and the avoidance of the costs of turnover. Planetree hospitals are often asked to quantify the incremental direct operating cost associated with adoption of the model. The capital costs associated with unit renovation to incorporate healing health care design principles and to create a healing environment vary widely from hospital to hospital but can be considerable. Normally, radical environmental changes are made when whole hospitals or hospital units are scheduled for replacement when they reach the end of their useful life. Planetree affiliates have proven that with creativity, attention to detail, and effective value engineering, a healing health care environment can be achieved with little or no construction premium.

The same can be said for labor costs. Richer nurse staffing ratios are rarely seen on Planetree units, and supplemental paid staff members are rarely incorporated. Most elements of the Planetree model are delivered by existing staff members or by the increased use of volunteers. The single biggest cost increase associated with the adoption of the model is staff training. However, the training costs never exceed 1 percent of operating costs, even for the most ambitious affiliate.

It is clear that the costs of implementing the Planetree model to an enlightened and highly motivated hospital are much less than the costs of maintaining the status quo. The value proposition has been demonstrated, and a requirement for such documentation should no longer deter the Planetree model from achieving its potential.

References

American Hospital Association Commission on Workforce for Hospitals and Health Systems. "In Our Hands: How Hospital Leaders Can Build a Thriving Workforce." April 2002.

Baker, S. K. *Managing Patient Expectations*. San Francisco: Jossey-Bass, 1998.

Ernst & Young LLP. *Built to Last Means Built to Change: Medicare+Choice and the New Health Care Consumerism*, June 1998.

Iacono, S. "Planetree Philosophy: A Study on the Relationship of Patient Satisfaction and Utilization of a Planetree Model in Care Delivery." *Plane Talk*, Sept./Oct. 2002, pp. 1–4.

Kavalier, F., and Spiegel, A. D. *Risk Management in Health Care Institutions*. Sudberry, Mass.: Jones and Bartlett, 1997.

Kohn, L. T., Corrigan, J., and Donaldson, M. S., *To Err Is Human: Building a Safer Health System*. Washington, D.C.: National Academies Press, 2000.

KPMG Peat Marwick LLP. "Consumerism in Health Care: New Voices." *Consumerism in Health Care Research Study Findings*, 1998.

Martin, D., and others. "Randomized Trial of a Patient-Centered Hospital Unit." *Patient Education and Counseling*, 1998, (34), pp. 125–133.

Pine, B. J., and Gilmore, J. *The Experience Economy*. Boston: Harvard Business School Press, 1999.

Press Ganey Associates. "One Million Patients Have Spoken: Who Will Listen?" *The Satisfaction Monitor*, 1999.

11

Creating Consensus
Partnering with Your Medical Staff

Steven Horowitz

In the vast majority of Planetree affiliate hospitals, as well as other patient-centered organizations, the local champions for the project are nurses. They perceive a patient-centered approach as the right way to treat patients. They are often joined by health care administrators who share this belief and have a vision of enhancing the image of the hospital within the community through patient advocacy. Surprisingly, physicians have rarely taken a leadership role in Planetree implementation around the country.

The mind-set of the physician has changed dramatically over the two decades of Planetree's existence. The rise of health maintenance organizations (HMOs), changing reimbursement strategies, and the political turbulence present in many financially challenged hospitals have had a dramatic impact on the psyche of practicing physicians. Unlike the earlier days of Planetree, when physicians were perceived as independent, entrepreneurial, and powerful, physicians have now joined nurses and other health care workers in their collective sense of disempowerment. As paperwork increases and reimbursement for medical services diminishes, there is a need for physicians to see more patients in less time in order to maintain the integrity of their practices. Thus, there is a growing sense of time urgency among physicians. These pressures have created a fundamental and philosophic conflict for physicians that strikes at the very heart and nature of medical practice. Physicians must either fall into line, spending less quality time with individual patients (and perhaps less time with their own families), or take home a smaller salary and risk marginalization by HMOs and medical centers that will view them as being less productive.

In the past, physicians held in the highest esteem by patients and the community because of their skill and compassion were therefore sought after as quality additions to the medical staff. At present, physicians with impossibly large practices based on complex business deals are the sought-after stars, with many of the traditional physician attributes taking a back seat to the hard reality of medical economics. Thus, depending on one's perspective, Planetree is either an outmoded, highly irrelevant "touchy-feely" concept that originated in San Francisco, or it is a concept needed now more than ever before, as physician and hospital priorities shift with the changing economic climate. The rapid increase in Planetree facilities around the country in recent years, broad media attention, and a growing interest in patient empowerment suggest that Planetree and similar concepts remain relevant to the evolution of the health care industry (Gearon, 2002).

Championing Patient-Centered Care

In general, physicians view Planetree as a positive change in the health care setting but often do not view establishment of a patient-centered culture as a high enough priority to champion the project, attend the retreats, or otherwise devote significant amounts of time to the program.

Full-time employees such as nurses and administrators participate in patient-centered activities, such as retreats and steering teams, "on hospital time," whereas physicians in private practice may lose income if they attend. In many cases, physicians question whether money spent on such "soft" modalities as patient education, art, and massage programs might not be better spent on a new x-ray machine

or an upgraded medical information system. Logically, full investment by all members of the health care team is more likely to result
in a seamless operation as perceived by patients and their family
members. Some Planetree hospitals require all staff members to participate in retreats and other Planetree-related informational sessions. It is a rare physician who does not already consider him- or
herself an expert on the subject of compassionate patient care, if only
there were enough time to practice that way on a consistent basis.
Unless required by hospital policy, physicians rarely choose to break
loose from their hectic schedules to participate in patient-centered
development and implementation activities.

A common malaise among health care workers in general and
physicians in particular relates to a perceived disparity between initial work expectations and the reality of the job at hand. In fact,
physicians have much to gain through participation in retreats and
other patient-centered activities, whether they involve other physicians exclusively or represent a vertically stratified cross-section of
the entire staff. In particular, Planetree retreats involving physicians
only, and led by a physician, offer an opportunity for more intimate
sharing of frustrations and they often open the door to physician-
inspired changes in patient care. Simply asking the question How
can you get closer to what you originally went into medicine for?
may start a more constructive dynamic for physicians initially interested only in venting their frustrations at a seemingly unresponsive
health care system. At the very least, physicians may be asked to
make individual commitments to changes in patient care that,
although small, may have a significant impact on the culture of the
hospital, in their aggregate. For instance, a physician may commit
to being a better listener or to arriving earlier at a clinic to avoid
having to rush through patients. In addition, the collective realiza-
tion at retreats that some problems can be addressed only by other
leadership groups within the hospital may be empowering for physicians by providing an outlet for their previously isolated voices.

Patient Access to Information

Not all Planetree concepts related to patient empowerment may be palatable to hospital-based physicians. Planetree originated as an educational library service prior to the first inpatient hospital unit in San Francisco, offering literature to patients in the form of packets of articles. This service provided information in the form of scientific papers, summary articles, and lay explanations, as well as information, at the patient's request, about complementary and alternative treatment options. The ability of the patient to participate in his or her treatment plan by asking informed questions or by choosing between different treatment strategies is fundamental to patient empowerment (Reiser, 1993; Vogel, 1993). However, free access to literature about more controversial forms of nonallopathic treatments is often problematic for physicians. For example, is it appropriate to have articles about chelation therapy within a hospital-based patient library when this is not considered a medically acceptable form of treatment? A conflict may exist between the conventional allopathic therapeutic community within the medical center and those who wish to provide free access to medically related information. The Planetree model is often mistakenly referred to as a form of alternative medicine. Since Planetree is about patient involvement and choice, it is not surprising that some patients will choose or ask questions about options not commonly found in many medical centers. Patients empowered to search for treatment strategies outside of those offered by the hospital may bring out an unintended conflict with physicians and administrators who do not believe in or use complementary modalities of treatment. Most Planetree hospitals provide options that fit within the culture of the institution and region. What "flies" in the Pacific Northwest may not be greeted so openly in the northeastern part of this country.

Complementary options such as acupuncture may be more acceptable in some medical centers because there is significant supportive

literature printed in standard medical journals, with potential usefulness described in the treatment of conditions such as low back pain
and the rehabilitation of the stroke patient. Other modalities, such
as healing touch, may be more controversial because of an absence of
supporting data, despite its benign nature. The implementation of
complementary therapeutic modalities is best done with careful sensitivity to the standard of care at each medical center. An aggres-
sive approach to using the Planetree model simply as a conduit to
introduce unproven alternative techniques will usually be counter-
productive and perceived as antagonistic by many physicians.

Physician Response to Open-Chart Policies

A similar difficulty has at times arisen from a related topic: the open-
chart policy that is common among Planetree affiliates. Although
most hospitals already provide access to medical records, it is unusual
for patients to have free access to their medical records while still
hospitalized. Some Planetree affiliates not only allow patients to read
their charts, they also permit patients to add their own comments,
although this option is rarely used by patients. Of course, the potential for a nurse's or physician's note saying, "Patient is doing well" to
be contradicted by an irate patient's note saying, "Like heck I'm
doing well, I feel terrible" strikes fear into the hearts of doctors,
administrators, and hospital lawyers. Paradoxically, there is evidence
that open charts may decrease the incidence of malpractice by
diminishing the patient's anxiety that critical information is being
intentionally withheld (Lichtstein, Materson, and Spicer, 1999). Just
the opportunity to read one's own chart may be enough to decrease
"serum paranoia" levels, even when the opportunity is not taken
advantage of by the patient. A reasonable concern about open charts
centers around the potential for misinterpretation by patients of written statements. For instance, a description of a dialysis patient having "end-stage renal disease" appearing in the chart of someone who
has been stable for years may cause unnecessary anxiety when read

by a patient unfamiliar with medical terminology. Toward this end, organizations may best offer free access to records with the assistance of a health care worker, who can be present to interpret statements or answer questions. It is equally essential that the medical staff be informed and on board with the policy, and that guidance be given regarding how progress notes might be clearly and tactfully written. This is a good strategy for reducing risk, regardless of whether an open-chart policy is in place.

Physician satisfaction surveys conducted in the original Planetree units in San Francisco and New York City suggested that doctors preferred Planetree units for their patients, compared with similar medical units elsewhere in the hospital (Blank, Horowitz, and Matza, 1995; Horowitz, 1995; Martin and others, 1998). Enhanced surroundings with a residential rather than institutional appearance, plus attention to the emotional well-being of patients and family members on Planetree floors, help to lessen the need for "apology rounds" by physicians. In addition, emotionally needy and depressed patients may benefit from ancillary programs provided by Planetree, such as massage, art, music, and relaxation therapy, when available. These programs add an additional dimension to patient care for stressed patients that may not be provided by time-strapped physicians, who may only spend a few minutes bedside (Roter and Hall, 1995; Fine, 1977).

At present, virtually all interpersonal interactions within an efficient hospital setting involve health care workers who take something *from* the patient (a history, blood) or do something *to* the patient (an ECG, an endoscopy). Units that use volunteer and care partner programs provide the patient with a trusting relationship within the hospital environment that involves someone who has no other motive than to provide emotional support and patient advocacy. A calmer, more secure, and informed patient is more likely to be better able to ask relevant questions and will be a better listener for physician responses. The physician-patient relationship still retains its own therapeutic value, and there is evidence that healing may occur more rapidly when patients are less stressed emotionally (Greenfield, Kaplan, and Ware, 1985; Kaplan, Greenfield, and Ware, 1989; Kiecolt-Glaser and others,1995).

An additional benefit of the Planetree approach for physicians who become involved through retreats and other functions is their discovery of other medical workers struggling with similar issues within the health care system. The ability to break through physician isolation and create bonds with other health care workers can be a powerful step toward authentic team building. While physicians tend to be the least actively involved members of the Planetree process, they are clearly indispensable members of the leadership team. A balanced approach that involves administration, nursing, and physician champions well attuned to the needs of patients and their families provides the best assurance that the evolution of the health care setting will not lose the essential elements of compassionate patient-centered care.

References

Blank, A. E., Horowitz, S. F., and Matza, D. L. "Quality with a Human Face? The Samuels Planetree Model Hospital Unit." *Journal of Quality Improvement*, 1995, *21*(6), 289–299.

Fine, V. K., and Thierren, M. E. "Empathy in the Doctor-Patient Relationship: Skill Training for Medical Students." *Journal of Medical Education*, 1977, *52*, 152–157.

Gearon, C. "Planetree." *Hospitals and Health Networks Magazine*, Oct. 2002, pp. 40–43.

Greenfield, S., Kaplan S., and Ware, J. E., Jr. "Expanding Patient Involvement in Care: Effects on Patient Outcomes." *Annals of Internal Medicine*, 1985, *102*, 520–528.

Horowitz, S. F. in K.W.M. Fulford, S. Eisser, and T. Hope (eds.), *The Planetree Model Hospital Project: Essential Practice in Patient-Centered Care*. Oxford, England: Blackwell Science, 1995.

Kaplan, S. H., Greenfield, S., and Ware, J. "Assessing the Effects of Physician-Patient Interactions on the Outcomes of Chronic Disease." *Medical Care*, 1989, *27* (supp. 3), 2110–2127.

Kiecolt-Glaser, J., and others. "Slowing of Wound Healing by Psychological Stress." *Lancet*, 1995, *346*(8984), 1194–1196.

Lichtstein, D., Materson, B., and Spicer, D. "Reducing the Risk of Malpractice Claims." *Hospital Practice*, 1999, 34(7), 69–72, 75–76, 79.

Martin, D., and others. "Randomized Trial of a Patient-Centered Hospital Unit." *Patient Education and Counseling*, 1998, (34), pp. 125–133.

Reiser, S. J. "The Era of the Patient: Using the Experience of Illness in Shaping the Missions of Health Care." *Journal of the American Medical Association*, 1993, *269*, 1012–1017.

Roter, D. L., and Hall, J. A. *Doctors Talking with Patients/Patients Talking with Doctors*. Westport, Conn.: Auburn House, 1995.

Vogel, D. "Patient-Focused Care." *American Journal of Hospital Pharmacology*, 1993, *50*, 2321–2329.

12

Recruitment and Retention

The Future of the Health Care Workforce

Charlene Honeycutt and Phyllis Stoneburner

The reality of health care is that no matter how much technology is invented or improved upon, or how many new drugs are created, it is still essentially about human beings caring for and nurturing other human beings. This premise is fundamental not only in the relationships between care providers and patients but equally so between care providers and the leaders of organizations that employ them. It is also critical in addressing not only today's issues with the health care workforce but also the future health of health care.

Recruitment and, more important, retention of compassionate and skilled employees are the highest priorities for health care organizations. The keys to success are firmly within our control.

Health Care Workforce Realities

According to the U.S. Department of Labor (2001), in its *Career Guide to Industries,* health services is one of the largest industries in the United States, with over eleven million jobs. Nine of the twenty occupations listed in the guide that are projected to grow the fastest will be in health services. Furthermore, the U.S. Department of Labor projects that 13 percent of all wage and salary jobs created between the years 2000 and 2010 will be in health services.

The shortage of health care workers represents a significant challenge both for the health care industry today and for the future—

but for two significantly different reasons. The current shortage is a result of increased demand for health care services. There are more practicing registered nurses, pharmacists, and other health care professionals than ever before in our nation's history. But, the increase in demand for health care services has been staggering. Emergency department visits are at an all-time high. The use of prescription drugs has increased, and so has life expectancy.

The shortage expected in the future is more ominous. In addition to a growing demand for services as the baby boomers age, the demographics of the current health care labor force will lead to more severe shortages. With the average age of nurses practicing in the United States at forty-five years and with declining school enrollments over the past several years, there will not be enough new nurses to replace those who retire or become disabled. It will be necessary to recruit more than one million workers into the health care professions to meet the projected future demand.

In October 1999, the Nursing Executive Center (1999), a division of the Advisory Board Company, based in Washington, D.C., published the results of a nationwide survey of registered nurses. The survey was designed not only to assess current issues and concerns for nurses but also to explore best practices that increase nursing satisfaction. The survey identified the following key employment attributes, listed in the order of importance:

1. Compensation

2. Scheduling options

3. Intensity of work

4. Competence of the clinical staff

5. Growth opportunities

6. Support services

7. Effectiveness of the direct manager

8. Participation in decision making

9. Recognition

The Nursing Executive Center's survey results have been sub-stantiated by a more recent national survey of registered nurses, con-ducted from October 2001 through March 2002 by Harris Interactive (2002) on behalf of *NurseWeek* and the American Orga-nization of Nurse Executives. The top issues identified in the sur-vey were better compensation, an improved work environment, better hours, and respect from management.

In addition, the North Carolina Center for Nursing released its findings from its 2001 survey of staff nurses in North Carolina (Lacey and Shaver, 2002). The findings noted that the same ele-ments were valued for both registered nurses and licensed practical nurses: "good compensation, positive collegial relationships, flexi-ble scheduling, and adequate staffing levels" (p. 12). These elements were found to be critical in all practice arenas: hospitals, long-term care facilities, and community nursing services.

Though the factors leading to nurse satisfaction have been the subject of intense scrutiny, the factors identified are not disparate from those that influence other clinicians. Findings from surveys of pharmacists, respiratory therapists, and radiology technicians all share the same themes: compensation, flexible scheduling, reward-ing practice environments, and effective communication with peers and leaders.

Current Best Practices

It is essential to evaluate and share best practices and opportunities for all health care practitioners, not only to recruit and retain cur-rent employees but also to benefit the entire industry.

Effectiveness of Direct Leadership and the
Critical Role of Communication

Excellent leadership in an organization has never been more essen-tial than it is today. Strategic planning, financial stewardship, and operational management have always been considered critical lead-ership skills. In today's workforce, however, it is the leader's people skills or emotional quotient that can make the difference in the organization's viability. Though once considered "soft" skills, communication and interpersonal relationship skills are now vital. Beverly Kaye and Sharon Jordan-Evans, in their book *Love 'Em or Lose 'Em: Getting Good People to Stay* (1999), state very simply that as a leader, "*you matter most*. . . . You actually have more power than anyone else to keep your best employees. Why? Because the factors that drive employee satisfaction and commitment are largely within your control" (p. 9).

The importance of leadership is clearly supported in research. In the Nursing Executive Center's national registered nurse survey, it was found that of those nurses dissatisfied with their direct leader, 84 percent had considered leaving the hospital. This was compared with nurses who were satisfied with their leaders, of whom only 43 percent had considered leaving. There is a high correlation between the leader's regard for the overall well-being of the staff and retention of staff members. This has always been a basic premise of the Planetree model: that health care is all about people taking care of people. Not only is it critical to provide kindness and care for patients, it is equally important for the leadership of an organization to do the same for the staff.

The role of the employees' direct leader is the most important one in an organization. In the past, especially in clinical departments in health care settings, people were promoted to leadership roles based on their clinical expertise. Though technical knowledge is important, it is not the only skill set needed to lead. In many organizations, short shrift has been given to developing communication skills. If any management training is provided, it is usually in conflict management. With little attention given to developing good communication skills, it is no surprise that conflict management courses are needed. Today's leaders need more thorough education and mentoring in people management—from the ability to communicate across intergenerational workforces to developing individual staff members and playing a key role in retention efforts.

Leadership has also been seen as systematic and rote, based on the notion that all employees need the same work and rewards to be motivated and productive. Timothy Butler and James Waldroop (1999) explore the art of leadership in retaining quality staff members. They define "job sculpting" as the ability of leaders to know their individual staff members and to understand what their interests are, what motivates them, and what brings them satisfaction. This knowledge allows the leader to match each employee with work that enables the employee to excel and thrive and increases the employee's commitment to the organization. The most essential job skill for leaders is the ability to listen—to what employees like and dislike in their jobs and what brings them joy and satisfaction on a day-to-day basis. Employees talk about these issues frequently. But are we listening?

With thought and creativity, job sculpting can be done at every level of the organization. It does not mean that people have to leave their clinical/operational environment or the bedside to excel. If there is a housekeeper who enjoys orienting others, that person could become a preceptor for new employees. A pharmacist who likes working with computers could take the lead in learning and troubleshooting the pharmacy's information systems. A nurse who enjoys working with data might assist with performance improvement activities. The complexity of our health care environment provides numerous opportunities to match individuals with work they find rewarding.

Job sculpting is only one aspect of an effective retention strategy. Another is to foster the role of *chief retention officer* in all supervisory staff members. For leaders to function as chief retention officers, organizations need to value skills such as coaching and mentoring as much as the ability to manage a budget.

Effectively leading a department requires the ability to perform periodic retention assessments. This assessment and intervention includes several important elements, beginning with staff participation in problem solving and brainstorming sessions to develop ideas for improvement. Not only does the staff's involvement assist with problem identification, it also provides an opportunity for participation in decision making. Staff members who are involved in creating the solutions are more closely aligned with the success of the outcome.

New Jersey's Hackensack University Medical Center, designated a magnet hospital by the American Nurses' Credentialing Center, involves staff members in their multidisciplinary councils. Hackensack's leadership is so committed to this process that they provide eight hours a month of paid time for those involved with the councils to attend meetings and complete the councils' work of improving the environment for patients and employees.

The retention assessment includes the development of department-specific metrics to track and trend. At Warren Memorial Hospital in Front Royal, Virginia, the nursing leaders maintain simple one-page, unit-specific dashboards that monitor nursing vacancy and turnover rates, patient satisfaction, the number of shifts covered by agency personnel, and the percentage of overdue performance appraisals. These dashboards are posted for the staff to review. Monthly monitoring allows the early identification of problem areas.

Leadership Style

An open-door leadership style that encourages staff members to express their concerns, views, and ideas is another important retention tool. This open-door approach includes consistent and thorough communication with the staff about hospital activities and decisions. This can be accomplished not only through face-to-face exchanges (both scheduled and spontaneous) but also through other avenues, such as electronic mail. Many Planetree facilities use both paper and electronic newsletters to facilitate communication. At Warren Memorial Hospital, this includes a monthly synopsis of the board of director's activities and decisions. This synopsis is e-mailed to the department leadership for sharing with the staff.

Open-door leadership also means going out to the staff, not just having the staff come to the leader. It encompasses leadership involvement in walking rounds to increase visibility, demonstrate interest, and provide opportunities to identify potential problems early. It also provides a forum for communication to enhance senior leadership's knowledge of each department's unique needs.

Employees are more likely to stay in an environment where they feel respected and valued, so providing recognition and feedback are critical elements for the chief retention officer. Both can be accomplished formally and informally. Recognition and celebration activities can focus on the individual employee, or they can be departmental or organization-wide. Recognition can be as simple as spoken feedback or handwritten notes to thank employees for specific acts. Griffin Hospital provides leaders with "toolboxes," which include items such as food, merchandise, and movie gift certificates and inspirational books and videotapes. These items can be used to spontaneously reward employees for excellent service. Griffin also formally recognizes individuals and departments with "best of the month" awards. Each quarter, Warren Memorial Hospital's leadership team cooks employee appreciation meals for all three shifts. Whatever the method, it is important for each leader to regularly communicate to employees how valuable they are to the organization.

Valley View Hospital created a newsletter that provides information about hospital activities, and it recognizes staff members for their dedication to quality care. Each issue includes updates about ongoing initiatives, and it celebrates the successes of their staff-driven work teams. A newsletter for physicians includes similar information.

An important tool for feedback is the performance appraisal, which should include both the technical aspects of a particular job and the organization's defined values. It is extremely important that performance appraisals be done in a timely manner, especially if the tool is tied to the compensation system. Performance appraisals should provide a balanced view of the employee, including both positive feedback and opportunities for improvement. Information provided at these meetings should never be a surprise to the employee. The performance appraisal is an opportunity to develop star performers. Once-a-year feedback, however, is not enough. Informal, frequent, and honest feedback needs to be provided to employees throughout the year.

But change is neither quick nor easy. Senior leaders must be committed to providing departmental leaders with the tools they need to serve as chief retention officers. Rigorous selection criteria are important for the leadership role; it is no longer enough to be technically competent. Roles must be clearly defined with appropriate compensation and incentives. Educational opportunities are vital, not only for new leaders but for seasoned ones as well. Feedback, coaching, and appropriate support should be ongoing. The organization must be committed to developing the chief retention officer role in every manager and supervisor.

Compensation

The issues around compensation are numerous and complex. How much is enough for each of the employee categories? How do we raise employees' salaries in times of shrinking reimbursement? How do we track accurate information about competitors' salaries in times when information sharing is taboo? How do we define who our competitors are? How often do we review and make changes?

One of the first steps needed is for management to define the compensation strategy for the organization. The strategy should address whether the organization wishes to be the market leader in salaries and benefits or be market-competitive. Guidelines should be developed regarding the frequency of changing salaries and benefits. Discussing these issues in advance allows the organization to proactively address compensation issues and to better articulate the strategy to employees.

A best practice recommended by the Nursing Executive Center is market-based compensation recalibration (H*Works, 2000). First, salary information is continually captured from a number of different sources: peer phone calls, employee exit interviews, newspaper and clinical journal advertisements, and formal self-accomplished or purchased salary surveys. This vigilance enables the organization to readily identify market trends.

A second component of the market-based compensation recalibration is a zip code analysis. The analysis looks at the zip codes of the clinical staff members employed at an organization to identify where staff members live and what facilities they pass as they come to work. The commuting pattern information helps to identify key competitors for labor.

The third component of market-based compensation recalibration is an ongoing assessment of how current strategies are working. This assessment can be as simple as a running time line with internal salary changes and turnover statistics tracked in tandem. The time line can also include other organizations' changes and the corresponding turnover in your own organization. These metrics allow the organization's leadership to make adjustments in compensation as needed.

It is important to communicate to staff the total value of their compensation and benefits. This can be accomplished by providing compensation and benefit fact sheets, or "road shows," to update the staff on a regular basis about the organization's compensation practices. The fact sheet can outline the rationale for changes, the dollar value of fringe benefits (a critical figure often overlooked by employees), and comparisons with other organizations. Also useful are compensation and benefit road shows—educational sessions in which staff members from Human Resources (HR) visit each department to answer questions. These sessions help to personalize information sharing and demonstrate that Human Resources department staff members are responsive to employee needs and concerns.

Using both written fact sheets and road shows combines two different mediums to appeal to the varied learning styles of a broad audience.

Scheduling and Work-Life Balance

Staff scheduling can be a challenge in any business, even those that do not operate twenty-four hours a day, seven days per week. Around-the-clock schedules coupled with on-call situations in operating rooms, maternity units, and other clinical and support service departments make hospital scheduling particularly difficult. In addition, the health care workforce remains predominantly female in nursing and is becoming predominantly female in the other clinical professions. For instance, the Bureau of Health Professions predicts that the pharmacy workforce, which was approximately 46 percent female in 2000, will be 58 percent female by 2010 (Health Resources and Services Administration, 2000).

To meet the needs of a health care workforce that is increasingly female, flexible scheduling options have begun to proliferate. Flexibility has become essential with shift lengths varying from four to eight, ten, and twelve hours. There are seven-on and seven-off scheduling patterns. Weekday versus weekend options are once again available in selected markets. Shift rotations vary from no rotation at all to rotations that are designed to better facilitate effective lifestyle patterns. What constitutes a "full-time" employee varies from 32 to 40 hours per week. In-house registries and float pools with more flexible schedules and higher salary and/or benefits are available. "Mom schedules," which take advantage of the times that children are in school (typically during the hours of 9 A.M. to 2 P.M.) have been successful in various practice settings. There are even models that allow employees to work nine months of the year, to correspond with their children's school year. The options are limited only by the creativity of the organization developing the schedules and the ability of the organization to absorb the increased operating cost that may result from less traditional schedules.

Best practices associated with scheduling revolve around creating and maintaining work-life balance and staff involvement in the scheduling process. Staff involvement in scheduling can vary from customized schedules, where the staff members request their ideal schedules and the final schedule is completed by the nursing leader, to self-scheduling, where staff members control the entire process. No matter what scheduling options are explored, flexibility is the key to success.

For optimum patient care, continuity must be maintained, especially when considering weekend versus weekday options. Continuity can be maintained in several ways: limiting the number of weekend-only positions, defining critical data elements that must be relayed between weekday and weekend staff members, and restructuring unit leadership roles (that is, of charge or resource nurses) to improve weekend support. These must be discussed and planned in advance to ensure that there is no difference in the level of care between one day of the week and another.

Fairness for all staff members must be addressed. The hospital's human resources department becomes a key partner in defining fair treatment standards and hiring practices for the staff. Fair treatment standards may require flexibility to meet the needs of individual departments. These standards should be clearly communicated to all staff members so that there are no surprises.

Conducting a scheduling gap analysis may also be helpful. This practice includes a comparison of the staff's preferred schedule to needed staffing levels. Once the gaps are identified, new staffing options and patterns can be explored. Hospital policies and procedures may need to be revised to support existing as well as new staffing patterns.

For organizations considering self-scheduling, there must be fair and consistent scheduling guidelines delineating specifics such as hours worked, maximum number of people off at a time, shift rotations (if required), weekend requirements, and vacation/holiday rotations. The staff must understand that unanticipated scheduling changes may still occur to meet the unit's, and ultimately the patients', needs. Units may create a staff council to address problems and resolve disputes.

Besides scheduling, work-life balance issues are also being addressed in innovative ways throughout the industry. For staff members who may be tired after working a twelve-hour shift and therefore not anxious to cook, some hospitals are providing take-home meals through the food service departments. Staff members can order from a select menu in the morning and pick up the meals as they leave the hospital. In addition, staples, such as bread and milk, can be purchased at the hospital, so that staff members needn't make an extra stop on the way home. Concierge services are being made available to the staff at some hospitals, including Warren Memorial. Necessary but time-consuming tasks, such as planning a vacation or sending a gift, can be accomplished via on-site or on-line concierge services. Concierge services can be offered via a hospital's own staff or through existing organizations that provide the service for a per-task or per-employee per-month fee.

Intensity of Work

Intensity of work issues are receiving nationwide attention. Most of this attention, both in the public press and with legislative bodies, has revolved around nurse-to-patient ratios and mandatory overtime. Intensity, however, is a reflection of far more than just those two issues. The health care workplace is increasingly complex; new technologies and medications emerge every day. Patient length of stay is short, so the work pace is fast and the paperwork continues to grow.

Unfortunately, there are no panaceas for these innumerable problems. Legislating staffing ratios and eliminating mandatory overtime will not provide a simple solution. However, by evaluating the issues that exist in organizations, solutions can be developed that will make a positive difference in the lives of employees.

Careful attention must be paid to evaluating, setting, and maintaining caregiver-to-patient ratios. Mandated ratios are not the answer. A new graduate may have difficulty handling a mandated ratio of one nurse to four patients, whereas an experienced nurse may be able to care for up to six patients. Each organization's administrative team, in concert with the clinicians who have a direct impact on patient care, must work together to define acceptable "do not exceed" limits. These limits should be evaluated and tested for both fiscal and clinical prudence. The limits must then be communicated to the staff with appropriate actions to take if the limits are breached. The actions might include closing beds, creating on-call schedules for high workload situations, and using internal float pools.

Work intensity can be monitored by using commercially available stress audits administered to the staff to help pinpoint sources of strain, such as the physical environment or the workload. It may also be helpful to have face-to-face meetings or focus groups with staff members to identify the top sources of stress for them. No matter what method is used, once stressors are identified, solutions can be found to reduce or eliminate them.

One stressor for nurses may be that a large number of admissions and discharges require an excessive time commitment. A targeted solution on high-volume units might be the creation of an admissions nurse—or even an admissions unit—that ensures that the immediate needs of admitted patients are met and that the nursing staff does not feel overwhelmed. A stressor for the pharmacy staff may be sharp peaks in the workload at certain times of day. Technology exists for medication order-entry to occur off-site; perhaps stay-at-home mothers or others who choose to work at home could be technologically connected to the hospital to assist at peak times. Other solutions for stress include offering employees chair massages, classes on stress management, and dedicated staff break rooms.

Competence of Clinical Staff and Growth Opportunities

Today's fast-paced clinical environments demand that all practitioners, even those newly hired, are ready to perform their jobs skillfully and efficiently. Two mechanisms to ensure the success of the staff's abilities are orientation and continuing education.

The orientation of new staff members to their work environment is an institution's investment both in its future and in the success of the employee. Unfortunately, orientation is often shortened
to save money. However, these cost "savings" often translate into
higher turnover and consequently higher costs. A well-planned and
well-executed orientation program is important not only for skill
development of new employees but also for the instilling of the
organization's philosophy and values.

Orientation need not be lengthy to be successful. However, it
must encompass some key elements, such as appropriate information for the practice arena, highly structured preceptorships (or
mentorships), frequent assessments of progress, and a continual
feedback loop.

Essential information elements for orientation should be defined
by both the leadership team and the staff in the department. This
should include both standard operating procedures and specific
required skill sets. The information can be disseminated in a variety of settings, both didactic and via preceptor at the bedside. One
model that is successful is to divide dissemination of essential information into "segmented" teaching, where didactic and bedside
teaching is interspersed. In the initial didactic activities, basic information, skills, and techniques are taught and practiced. These initial classes are followed by the structured provision of care under
supervision on the units for low- to moderate-risk patients. After a
defined interval, the employee returns to the classroom setting for
more advanced information and skill practice. This is again followed
by structured clinical experiences with high-risk patients. This cycle
allows the new employee time to process information and skills at
the basic level first and then to grow, once proficiency is demonstrated. This allows employees the time to assimilate information
and build self-confidence.

No matter whether the employee is new or experienced, a preceptor or mentor is important. Mentoring is an important tool in
improving communication, reducing frustration, and improving the

overall delivery of patient care. Preceptors should be role models in terms of their care philosophy, desired behaviors, organizational values, and clinical and teaching skills. This role is so significant that many institutions have an application process for selecting preceptors. It is also important to ensure that preceptors are knowledgeable about adult education principles, goal setting, providing constructive feedback, and letting go when the time is right. A preceptor for each new employee should be selected, based on compatibility and the outlined needs of the new employee. Once this has occurred, the orientation plan, including goals to be met, can be formalized.

Frequent assessments of the orientation process should be made periodically by the preceptor and orientee to review procedures and ensure that orientation needs are being met. In addition, weekly progress should be evaluated. This allows problems to be recognized early and course corrections to be made, if required.

This progress assessment not only identifies individual issues, it also provides the organization with continual feedback on the success of the overall orientation program. If problems or issues are identified that affect multiple departments (such as issues related to intravenous therapy), that part of the orientation can be reevaluated and changed. Changes may be as simple as conducting a more thorough review of a policy or meeting the need for the development of a mock code-blue session.

The University of North Carolina Health Care System has encompassed many of these best practices in its Critical Care Odyssey Nursing Residency Program. Mary Hall, director of internships, describes the process as providing not only the information needed for new employees to perform their new roles but also establishing links and networks necessary to create supportive and nurturing social networks. For a new critical care nurse, the experience starts with a weeklong general orientation to the hospital and nursing department, including providing typical information about nursing policies and procedures, infection control, and clinical information systems. This is followed by what makes their program unique—a one-week "boot camp," complete with identification dog tags. Boot camp is designed to develop essential critical care skills (such as arrhythmia analysis and advanced cardiac life support) as well as the tools to develop critical thinking skills and nursing judgment. Boot camp also encompasses care at the end of life and how to care for caregivers. Equally important is that boot camp begins the socialization and peer group formation that is critical to a new employee's success. The week of boot camp culminates in a graduation ceremony, where each new employee receives a diploma as well as a set of business cards. Employees' families are encouraged to attend the ceremonies, as it provides an opportunity for family members to learn more about the health care setting.

Boot camp is followed by Phase I of a formal preceptorship, where the new employee is paired with an experienced staff member for a period of six weeks. During Phase I, the orientee is not included in the staffing count. Phase II is an additional six-week period, during which the new employee is counted in the staffing mix but has the support of an assigned "resource" nurse. After the first six to eight months, a benchmark test for competency is given to assess the employees' progress and needs. The tests are designed specifically for the critical care units in which the employees work.

An additional component of the Critical Care Odyssey Nursing Residency Program is its ongoing support for the first year of employment, through a series of monthly luncheon lectures. The topics covered vary, based on feedback from the new staff members and the needs assessed by the leadership group.

At the end of the first year of employment, a candle lighting ceremony is held to celebrate the successes of the employees. This ceremony is also a mechanism for the leadership to thank the employees for their hard work and dedication. After the first year of this structured orientation program, there was only a 3 percent attrition rate. Because of the success of this program, the model has also been incorporated into women's services and children's services, and will soon be incorporated into medical-surgical oncology.

In addition to having a good orientation program in place, it is critical to offer opportunities for educational advancement to tenured staff members. Ongoing education not only encourages individuals' growth, it also ensures that the organization continues to improve its performance. The traditional mechanism for education has been department-based in-service sessions. However, new information technologies provide additional ways to educate, such as computer-based tutorials that present practical situations to test critical thinking skills and demonstrate real-time results. The Internet's growth has led to the creation of multiple on-line educational services, enabling employees to attend classes from their own homes. Tuition reimbursement programs, coupled with service back to the organization as "repayment," can be an important retention tool. Because of the breadth of these new services, educational opportunities can be provided to employees at varying degrees of cost.

Mid-Columbia Medical Center (MCMC) in The Dalles, Oregon, brought all of its orientation and education programs together to create the MCMC University. Instilling the values and goals of the organization is considered to be as important as skill building and personal development. An orientation for new staff members focuses on team building, attitudes, innovation, quality, and the providing of great service. Annual staff retreats for all departments reemphasize values and provide opportunities for staff input.

The Future

Attracting people to health care careers needs to start early. Many institutions have created coloring books for young children that not only showcase health careers but also promote positive health habits. These are distributed at school career days and parent events, as well as when children access health care arenas (such as when they make trips to the emergency department). Many orga-nizations organize tours so that children can see the hospital in a fun, nonthreatening fashion, often giving away masks and hair cov-ers as part of the tour.

School- and hospital-sponsored organizations, such as Future Nurses of America, are returning. There are innovative programs for groups, such as the Girl Scouts of the USA, that provide merit badges for exploring health careers. Pennsylvania's and North Car-olina's Nursing Exploration Patch, available to Junior, Cadette, and Senior Girl Scouts, is an excellent example of this. The goal of these programs is to increase exposure to the health professions—notably the incredible variety of options, the educational diversity, and the tremendous need.

In addition, health care organizations must also educate school career counselors about the wide variety of health care options. Pro-viding counselors with educational and shadowing experiences in the hospital allows them to experience the importance and diver-sity of health care roles.

Start Now

Johnson and Johnson Health Care Systems, Inc. proved to be a tremendous partner in health care recruitment when it unveiled its $20 million multiyear initiative called The Campaign for Nursing's Future. This campaign includes "I'm a Nurse" and "They Dare to Care" television advertisements, coupled with the Discover Nursing Web site (http://www.discovernursing.com). These portray nursing as the exciting, fulfilling career that it is through the eyes of prac-ticing nurses. The nurses showcased represent not only the variety of opportunities but also the diverse participants in nursing. In addi-tion, the campaign includes scholarship funds. This unprecedented move has created a new way to encourage nursing as a career choice.

Unique partnerships have been created in communities across the country. Schools offering education and training in health care careers have developed partnerships with hospitals for financial and clinical support. Hospitals, such as Warren Memorial, have partnered with high schools to teach credit-based curricula for both certified nursing assistants and licensed practical nurses (LPN). These programs enable students to sit for their nursing assistant certification examination by the eleventh grade and their LPN examination at the completion of high school.

Competing hospitals have banded together to provide community-wide educational sessions on health care, partnering with the local Chamber of Commerce. Internship programs—collaborative efforts among high schools, colleges, and hospitals—have been created to provide both didactic and skills training sessions (in such areas as cardiopulmonary resuscitation, mock surgeries, and lifting and transfer techniques) in hospital settings, to expose students to the real world of health care. Scholarships have been created for students to attend school, with future repayment being in the form of their employment. The government has increased its financial support in the form of school loan repayment for working in underserved communities. The government has unveiled a new on-line clearinghouse (http://www.CareCareers.net) that is dedicated exclusively to those seeking careers in the long-term care arena.

Options exist for bringing nurses back into the field, including refresher courses for nurses who have not practiced in years. These courses are often paid for by the hospitals, in return for a work commitment. The intent of the program is to reeducate nurses and develop the skills they will need in today's environment. In a similar program, Virginia's Williamsburg Community Hospital has developed special opportunities for retired nurses to volunteer as care partners for patients who do not have family members to function in this role. Retired nurses can choose their schedule, which may be just four hours per week, and a special orientation is held for them. They are then deployed to patient care floors to assist with routine care tasks, such as wound dressing changes, tube feedings, and ambulation, as well as providing comfort measures, such as brewing a cup of tea or engaging in good conversation.

Look to Technology

Continued changes in technology will play a key role in the health care of the future by supporting the delivery of better and more productive care. The technology already exists for pharmacists to input orders from their own homes. Beds are available that convert from sleeping surfaces to chairs to standing positions, eliminating the potential for back injuries in staff members. Integration of health care devices and clinical documentation systems will eliminate the need for manual documentation and the redundancies that exist today. Mobile communication devices will allow more freedom for the staff. The future possibilities are incredible.

Increase Minority Representation in Health Care

The importance of diversity needs to be recognized so as to increase minority and ethnic representation in all health professions. Demographics in the United States are changing significantly, but this has not been reflected in the health care workforce. The pool of talent extends far beyond what has been embraced to date.

South Carolina's Greenville Hospital System has taken the lead in improving diversity representation in health care. Fred Hobby, Greenville's chief diversity officer, notes that increasing minority and ethnic representation in health care is a multifactorial process, starting with commitment from the organization's leadership to either groom and grow from within the organization's ranks or recruit from outside. This commitment also includes an assessment of the organization's internal structure and whether the makeup of the senior administrative team resembles the community served. Hobby notes that recruitment and retention are enhanced if the leadership team is representative of the community.

It is also important to evaluate the recruitment process for its sensitivity to the cultural needs of the potential employee. Hobby states that the best recruiter for a minority is another minority. This provides not only an introduction to the organization but also the development of social and community connections.

Because a sense of isolation can be detrimental to both recruitment and long-term retention, it is critical for an organization to create an environment where there is a sense of belonging, both personally and professionally.

Greenville Hospital System has also partnered with a local college to provide educational opportunities for those interested in becoming patient care technicians. The hospital financially sponsors students for both the course fees and child care. The college holds the courses off campus in various community settings to allow people opportunities to attend closer to their homes. This hospital-community partnership has increased Greenville's ability to reach out to more minorities who are interested in working in health care.

A comprehensive assessment must be performed to understand the barriers that limit minority representation. Language, educational, and financial barriers must be identified and addressed. Recruitment opportunities need to extend beyond the traditional educational settings, going into churches and social settings. It will take the focused actions not only of federal and state governments but also of local communities to ensure that their systems represent the community and meet the needs of their constituents.

Summary

No doubt, new challenges to recruiting and retaining an adequate health care workforce will be uncovered over the course of time. Fortunately, attention generated by the current shortages has resulted in the development and implementation of a variety of innovative strategies that it is hoped will bear fruit in both the short and long terms.

References

Butler, T., and Waldroop, J. "Job Sculpting: The Art of Retaining Your Best People." *Harvard Business Review*, Sep./Oct. 1999, pp. 144–152.

Harris Interactive. "NurseWeek/AONE Survey." *NurseWeek*, 2002. [http:www.nurseweek.com/survey/summary_print.html].

Health Resources and Services Administration. *The Pharmacist Workforce: A Study of the Supply and Demand for Pharmacists*. Rockville, Md.: Health Resources and Services Administration, 2000.

H*Works. *Reversing the Flight of Talent—Best Practices for Attracting and Retaining Nursing Talent*. Washington, D.C.: Advisory Board Company, 2000.

Kaye, B., and Jordan-Evans, S. *Love 'Em or Lose 'Em: Getting Good People to Stay*. San Francisco: Berrett-Koehler, 1999.

Lacey, L. M., and Shaver, K. "Retaining Staff Nurses in North Carolina." Unpublished research paper, The North Carolina Center for Nursing, 2002.

Nursing Executive Center. *Nursing Executive Center National RN Survey*. Washington, D.C.: Advisory Board Company, 1999.

U.S. Department of Labor. *Career Guide to Industries*. Washington, D.C.: U.S. Department of Labor, Bureau of Labor Statistics, 2001.

13

Green Hospitals

The New Health Care Environmentalism

Trevor Hancock

There has been growing concern over the past thirty years—since the first U.N. conference on the environment, held in Stockholm in 1972—with the environmental impacts of our industrialized society and with the human health effects of such impacts. Those impacts include

- Climate and atmospheric changes, including global warming, the depletion of the ozone layer, acid rain, and urban air pollution

- Air, water, and soil pollution and the contamination of food chains and ecosystems with persistent organic pollutants, heavy metals, and other toxic substances

- Depletion of renewable resources such as fisheries, topsoil, forests, and freshwater, as well as of such nonrenewable resources as fossil fuels

- Destruction of habitat, reduction of biodiversity, and growing human-induced mass extinction of species, all of which result in the fraying of the web of life

The overall result is a disruption of ecosystem stability and an impairment of ecosystem health that is threatening the very underpinnings of our global life support systems, our economies, our societies, and our health (Hancock and Davies, 1997).

In response to these concerns, we have seen a growing interest in sustainable development and in the "greening" of our activities. The Dow Jones Index now includes a sustainability index, and the business world is abuzz with interest in such concepts as *nature's economy* and *natural capital* (Hawken, Lovins, and Lovins, 1999), while pension and mutual funds that include companies that meet established criteria for sustainability are proving to be profitable.

In recent years, this issue has begun to receive attention in the health care system. It is increasingly being recognized that health care—which in 2000 was a $1.3 trillion industry, or 13.2 percent of the entire U.S. gross domestic product (GDP), with projected growth to $2.8 trillion, or 17 percent of GDP, by 2011 (Centers for Medicare and Medicaid Services, 2002)—has a very large environmental impact. As a general rule, there are human health impacts associated with those environmental impacts. This means that the health care system, in providing health care, may also be harming the health of people, not only locally but indeed globally. But this is incompatible with a fundamental ethical precept of health care, embedded in the Hippocratic Oath, which is to *do no harm*, as the U.S.-based international coalition Health Care Without Harm has pointed out. Thus the health care system has an ethical duty to minimize its environmental and human health impact and to behave in an environmentally responsible manner—to become more "green."

The health care system as a whole, and the hospital in particular, is a potent symbol of health to its community. As such, health care facilities should strive to be role models of environmentally responsible practices. It is ironic that the health care system, which frequently includes in its mission statement the promotion of the health of the community, has been identified by the U.S. Environmental Protection Agency (EPA) as a significant source of both dioxin pollution (as a result of the incineration of polyvinyl chloride (PVC) and other chlorinated products) and mercury pollution. Hospitals and other health care facilities are also important contributors to both air pollution and greenhouse gas emissions because of their above-average use of energy, their significant consumption of a variety of resources, their use of toxic chemicals such as pesticides, and their production of solid, liquid, and gaseous wastes.

Planetree hospitals have always paid great attention to the impact of the environment on patients, visitors, and staff members alike. From its earliest beginnings, the Planetree approach has placed strong emphasis on the quality of the environment within the hospital walls. Indeed, there has often been an effort to naturalize the indoor environment through the use of plants, fish tanks, fountains, pet visitation, and even waterfalls. There has also been an effort to connect the indoor environment with the outdoor environment by providing views to attractive outdoor settings. Planetree hospitals also stress the importance of healing gardens and similar restful spaces for patients, family members, and staff members as part of the milieu of a healing environment and a healthy workplace.

Not only should Planetree hospitals be concerned about how the environment affects the provision of health care and the quality of the healing experience; they also have to be concerned about how the provision of health care affects the environment. With their commitment to excellence and leadership, such a task is entirely consistent with the philosophical approach of hospitals in the Planetree Alliance.

How Health Care Adversely Affects the Environment and Human Health

The health care system contributes to environmental harm through its use of resources and its production of wastes. Four broad issues lie at the heart of health care's environmental impact: energy use, the consumption of other resources, the use of toxic materials, and the production of waste—in particular solid waste and toxic emissions and effluents.

Energy Use and Its Health Impacts

"If hospitals improved their energy efficiency by an average of 30 percent, the annual electricity savings would be nearly $1 billion and 11 million fewer tons of carbon dioxide would be emitted—equivalent to taking 2 million cars off the road" (Whitman, 2001).

The first issue that hospitals need to address is their use of energy, since energy use makes up roughly half of the total ecological footprint of buildings (Wackernagel and Rees, 1996). The ecological footprint provides an integrative method for assessing the overall impact of an activity, facility, community, or nation in terms of the amount of land required to produce the resources that are consumed or absorb the wastes that are produced. In the only assessment of the ecological footprint of a hospital yet carried out, energy use represented up to 80 percent of the ecological footprint (Germain, 2002).

As one might expect, North American hospitals are particularly profligate in their energy use. In a comparison of electrical and thermal energy consumption for typical hospitals in nine countries (Centre for the Analysis and Dissemination of Demonstrated Energy Technologies, 1997), Canada and the United States stand out as having the highest average annual electrical consumption/m^2 of gross floor area and the highest average annual thermal energy consumption, respectively.

According to the U.S. Department of Energy's Energy Information Administration (2002), although health care buildings in the United States are among the least prevalent type of commercial building, at 2.3 percent, they account for 11 percent of all commercial energy consumption. In Canada, in 1997, the health sector also accounted for 11 percent of the energy used in the commercial and institutional sector (Natural Resources Canada, 2000).

In addition, the construction, supplying, and maintenance of the health care system requires a significant share of the activity of the transportation and industrial sectors as well, which between them account for more than 65 percent of energy use in Canada. So the total energy use by the health care system, directly and indirectly, is substantial.

The environmental and health impacts of energy use are very large. They include the health impact of prospecting for, extracting, transporting, refining, processing, producing, and distributing all forms of energy prior to their use, as well as the subsequent impact of waste disposal and the decommissioning of energy plants (Romm and Ervin, 1996).

Of particular concern is the use of fossil fuels, since they contribute to such important environmental and health effects as global warming and air pollution. The health care system uses fossil fuels both directly—for such things as space and water heating, steam generation, vehicle use, and on-site incineration—and indirectly—through its use of electrical energy from fossil fuel–fired plants, energy for the production of construction materials, products and services used by the health care system, and fossil fuel for transportation of the people and goods needed to operate the health care system.

The environmental and health impacts of greenhouse gas emissions and the associated global warming have been the topic of extensive research and discussion in recent years (Intergovernmental Panel on Climate Change, 1996; McMichael and others, 1996; McCarthy and others, 2001). The environmental impacts include such massive changes as the melting of glaciers and continental ice caps, an increased sea level, major changes in wind and ocean currents, the melting of permafrost, and major shifts in natural and agricultural ecosystems.

The health impacts are both direct and indirect and will occur not just in North America but globally. Direct health impacts will include more disease and deaths from heat waves and the worsening air pollution likely to accompany higher urban temperatures, as well as disease and deaths resulting from an increase in severe weather events. These health effects will occur globally, but of particular concern is the potential for flooding and storm surges in low-lying delta areas, such as the Bay of Bengal, where millions may be affected.

The larger health impacts are likely to be indirect. They include the wider dispersion of the insect vectors of a number of infectious diseases. Of particular concern is the anticipated increase in malaria worldwide as malarial mosquitoes are able to survive and breed further north and south and at higher altitudes. In North America, there is concern about increased exposure to such conditions as the West Nile virus, dengue fever, and Lyme disease. Even more massive health impacts may result from changes in agricultural ecosystems, which may lead to the displacement of large populations around the world, with the attendant health effects of mass migration and refugee conditions.

Fossil fuel combustion also results in air pollution, which has significant impacts on both mortality and morbidity. Through the use of fossil fuels, especially for the generation of electricity, the health care system contributes to air pollution and thus to disease and death in the community. One estimate is that up to seven hundred thousand lives a year could be saved worldwide as a result of lower levels of air pollution (World Resources Institute, 1998). A recent report on the illness costs of air pollution in Ontario, Canada, notes that for every death there are 5.1 hospital admissions, 6.8 emergency room visits, and 24,128 minor illness days (Ontario Medical Association, 2000). Although the health care system is clearly not the principal source of such health-damaging air pollution, the fact that it contributes at all to this significant health problem is a cause for concern.

Resource Use

The construction and operation of hospitals consumes vast amounts of resources. Building construction also generates significant waste. It is estimated that 25 to 40 percent of municipal solid waste is from construction and demolition alone. The health care industry in the United States builds some seventy to seventy-five million square feet of space each year (Weinhold, 2001).

In their ongoing operations, hospitals use large amounts of paper and plastics, as well as glass, wood, and metal. This results in part from a concern with infection control, so that many single-use, disposable products are used. But the "disposable mentality," common everywhere in society and perhaps heightened in hospitals by their unique concerns about infection control, may often extend well beyond real need to a pattern of behavior based on convenience. The extensive use of paper and plastics has implications for the sustainability of both a key renewable source (forests) and a key nonrenewable resource (oil), not to mention the need to reduce disposal costs.

An indication of the scale of such resource use comes from the estimation of the ecological footprint of the Lion's Gate Hospital in North Vancouver, British Columbia (Germain, 2002). In this 580-bed community hospital (with roughly half the beds being used for chronic care),

- More than 1.75 million pairs of gloves were used in the course of one year, or 8.2 pairs per patient per day, 98 percent of them being nonsterile gloves for patient care

- More than 135,000 adult disposable diapers and more than 31,000 disposable incontinence pads were used

- It was estimated that almost 220 tons of paper were brought into the hospital

The health effects of the consumption of these and other resources is, like energy use, associated with the life cycle costs of their use, from initial extraction to final disposal. Whether the resource is renewable (forest products such as wood and paper, freshwater, natural fibers such as cotton, or all sorts of food) or nonrenewable (metals, and minerals, and plastics from oil), there are both environmental impacts and related health impacts arising from their use (Hancock and Davies, 1997). A broader concern is that the depletion of these resources may threaten the livelihood, health, and well-being of populations remote from us geographically (South American forest dwellers, fishermen in Asia, and so forth) or remote from us in time (our descendants).

Use and Disposal of Toxic Substances

The health care system uses a wide variety of toxic substances in its day-to-day operations. Of particular concern are cleaning agents, disinfectants, and pesticides, as well as laboratory chemicals, pharmaceutical products, and radioactive materials. In addition, and of growing concern, is the problem of dioxin production and mercury pollution as a result of the incineration of medical wastes.

Cleaning products include floor buffers, floor strippers, glass cleaners, carpet cleaners, metal cleaners, solvents, and degreasers, whereas disinfectants include quaternary ammonium compounds, phenols, chlorine, alcohols, aldehydes, and oxides (Homer, 2001). Their use can affect the quality of freshwater and groundwater and can increase health risks to fish and other wildlife. Other environmental problems associated with cleaning agents include the contamination of food chains and air pollution, and the human health problems that may result include respiratory sensitivity, skin irritation or allergy, contact dermatitis, and asthma.

Hospitals use a wide variety of toxic laboratory materials, some of which have to be collected and disposed of as hazardous waste and some of which are discharged in wastewater effluents. As a result, wastewater effluents may contain low concentrations of such chemicals as nickel, copper, zinc, silver, mercury, cyanide, phenolic compounds, solvents, glutaraldehyde, and formaldehyde (Canadian Centre for Pollution Prevention and Broadhurst Environmental Management, Inc., 1996). Mercury, for example, is found in a wide variety of chemicals used in the laboratory, particularly as histology fixatives and stains, and it is also found in antiseptics and preservatives, as well as in batteries (Environment Canada, Ontario Region, n.d.). Given the large volume of effluents, the total loading of such chemicals into the environment may be quite large.

In addition, hospitals often also use a number of different pesticides. In a 1995 report on pest management in New York state hospitals, the office of New York's attorney general found that thirty-three active pesticide ingredients were applied in virtually all areas of most of the hospitals throughout the state; indeed, the report found that 98 percent of hospitals use pesticides. Given the potential harm that pesticides can cause, this is somewhat troubling, particularly since they found that in the vast majority of cases, pesticides were used routinely, not in response to a specific problem. Even worse, they also found that written notice was not provided to patients and employees regarding pesticide use in more than half of the hospitals. Even though the report recommended reducing pesticide use, in particular through integrated pest management, Weinhold (2001) comments that "little action on the issue, in New York hospitals or elsewhere around the country, has since occurred."

Another class of toxic materials that is attracting growing attention is pharmaceuticals. Pharmaceuticals may end up in the solid or liquid waste stream, either because they are placed there on purpose or through secretion in urine or feces. Among the most toxic are cytotoxic drugs, which have to be treated as biomedical waste (Canadian Centre for Pollution Prevention and Broadhurst Environmental Management, Inc., 1996). These concerns have long been recognized, but recent concern has begun to focus on the more subtle impact of pharmaceuticals and personal care products on the environment. A review by Daughton and Ternes (1999) notes that these products, which include both human and veterinary prescription drugs, diagnostic agents, fragrances, and sunscreen agents, "can continually be introduced to the aquatic environment as complex mixtures via a number of routes, but primarily by both untreated and treated sewage" (p. 907). They note that very little is known about the effects of these products on aquatic or terrestrial

life, although we do know that "these substances have the potential to be profoundly bioactive."

Among the pharmaceuticals of concern are antibiotics, antide-
pressants, hormones, and many other drugs that may have subtle
effects on behavior, reproductive, and developmental outcomes in
a range of aquatic organisms. Daughton and Ternes note a German
study that looked only at aspirin, paracetamol, clofribric acid (a
blood lipid regulator), and methotrexate. The study states that
"unmetabolized, the loading of these drugs into bodies of water in
Germany could be hundreds of tons per year" (Henschel, Wenzel,
Diedrich, and Fliedner, 1997).

Finally, hospitals use a variety of radioactive materials in both
diagnostic and therapeutic activities. The safe use and disposal of
these materials is subject to federal regulation; a green health care
strategy would seek to minimize the need for such materials.

Medical Waste Incineration

There has been growing concern about the environmental and
health impact of medical waste incineration, which can be a source
of a number of pollutants, including particulate matter and two key
toxic substances: dioxins and mercury.

Dioxin is the most potent human carcinogen known. One
important source is the incineration of hospital wastes that
includes PVC and other plastics. The high chlorine content of
PVC (up to 50 percent by weight) makes it an important factor
in the generation of dioxins and other polychlorinated organic
compounds in situations where incineration occurs at lower temperatures, as is the case in older incinerators (Health Care Without Harm, 2001). PVC is also a concern because of the use of
DEHP, a plasticiser, in IV bags and tubing. Concern has been raised
about the health effects, particularly for neonates (Health Care
Without Harm, 2002).

Mercury is a known neurotoxin that accumulates in the food
chain.

In the United States, "medical waste incineration has been identified by the EPA as the third largest known source of dioxin air emissions[, whereas] an estimated ten percent of the mercury emissions to the environment from human activities comes from medical waste incineration" (Health Care Without Harm, 2001). See "Background on Incineration" at http://www.noharm.org/index.cfm?page_ED=11.[1]

Solid Waste Production

Health Care Without Harm (1998) reported that the volume of waste produced by hospitals in the United States per bed had more than doubled since 1955. It was estimated that hospitals produced 7 kilograms of waste per bed per day, due primarily to the increased use of plastics and disposables, unnecessary biohazard disposal, and inefficient waste management. A 1990 audit of the Ottawa General Hospital in Ontario, Canada, found that the composition of the 5.5 kg/bed/day of waste that was produced was

- 45 percent—paper

- 17 percent—food

- 14 percent—plastic

- 6 percent—liquids

- 5 percent—biomedical

- 5 percent—miscellaneous

- 3 percent—glass

- 3 percent—wood

- 2 percent—metal (Canadian Centre for Pollution Prevention and Broadhurst Environmental Management, Inc., 1996)

Tieszen and Gruenberg's study (1992) examined the composition of surgical waste from five different sorts of surgical procedures in a tertiary teaching hospital in Michigan. A total of 274.7 kilograms of surgical waste arising from twenty-seven cases was examined and the composition was as follows:

- 39 percent—disposable linens

- 26 percent—plastic

- 7 percent—paper

- 27 percent—miscellaneous waste

Disposable linen, paper, and recyclable plastic accounted for 73 percent by weight and 93 percent by volume of the total surgical waste. When extrapolated to a national level for the United States, it was estimated that these five types of procedures alone would generate annually twenty-three million kilograms of waste occupying approximately four hundred thousand cubic meters of space. The authors estimated that by using reusable linen products and engaging in currently available and feasible recycling methods, the weight of surgical waste nationally could be substantially reduced.

Most of the solid waste produced by the health care system can safely go to landfill. However, Health Care Without Harm (1998) points out that in the United States, anywhere from 75 to 100 percent of medical waste is incinerated, even though only 10 to 15 percent of hospital waste is infectious, and only 1 to 2 percent of medical waste actually needs incineration to protect the health of the public.

Overall Impact

Some sense of the scale of the environmental impact of the health care system can be gained from the economic input-output life cycle assessment method developed by researchers at the Green

Design Initiative of Carnegie Mellon University. Using data from the U.S. Department of Commerce, this site (http://www.eiolca.net) makes it possible to estimate the overall economic, environmental, and health and safety impact of—among other things—the health care system. For any given dollar amount of services provided, the model quantifies the impact for the entire supply chain of requirements. In the case of hospitals, producing one million dollars' worth of health care services (and it is worth remembering that the health care industry in the United States in 2000 was a $1.3 trillion industry, of which 32 percent, or $416 billion, was attributable to hospitals [Centers for Medicare & Medicaid Services, 2002]) involves the use of over 250,000 kilowatt-hours of electricity, 41 metric tons of ores, 161 metric tons of fuel, and over two million gallons of water, as well as the release of the equivalent of 430 metric tons of carbon dioxide, 4.7 metric tons of conventional pollutants, and almost one-third of a metric ton of toxic releases and transfers (Green Design Initiative, 2000). The total environmental impact of the hospital sector can be assumed to be roughly 416,000 times greater.

Unfortunately, not only has there been no overall assessment of the environmental impact of health care, but there has not yet been a comprehensive environmental impact assessment of even an individual hospital. The nearest we have come to this, so far, is an assessment of the ecological footprint of the Lion's Gate Hospital (Germain, 2002), the first time that such an assessment has ever been carried out. The ecological footprint of Lion's Gate Hospital, with an average daily inpatient count of 591 patients, of whom approximately 280 were extended care residents, was 2,841 hectares, or 4.81 hectares per patient per year. This is compared with the average Canadian ecological footprint of 7.66 hectares per person. Given the area of the hospital site (3.95 hectares), the hospital's ecological footprint is more than seven hundred times its actual size. This is compared with the ecological footprint of the city of Vancouver, which is approximately 180 times that of its "political area."

Another aspect of the overall environmental impact on hospitals themselves is the direct and indirect costs, which are likely to be quite high. For example:

- Inefficient use of energy leads to ongoing costs that, in the long run, often exceed the costs of improving existing buildings and operating procedures, or designing new, energy-efficient buildings.

- Single-use, disposable products may seem cheaper at the point of purchase but not when disposal costs are factored in.

- Costs per ton for incineration of waste are higher than for normal solid waste disposal.

- Good recycling programs have the potential of generating revenue.

- The use of or emitting chemicals that are less environmentally and occupationally harmful may be cheaper than the safe handling and disposal of cheaper but more toxic chemicals.

- Improper handling and disposal of toxic chemicals may open up hospitals to prosecution resulting in fines under state or federal laws.

Finally, and perhaps of greatest importance to the health care system, arising from the environmental impact of the health care system there is an impact on human health. This puts the system in conflict with its underlying ethical precept of doing no harm. A full health impact assessment of the environmental damage resulting from the health care system's activities must await the assessment of the health care system's overall environmental impact. However, given that the health care system is about 14 percent of the

American economy, it is quite clear that the impact is likely to be quite significant. Some of the ways in which the health care system's environmental impact may well contribute to mortality and morbidity include

- Respiratory and cardiovascular disease and premature death associated with air pollution

- Potentially massive long-term health effects resulting from global warming

- Health effects resulting from the dispersion of dioxin, mercury, and other contaminants into the environment and the food chain

- Health effects for staff and patients resulting from the use of pesticides and other toxic materials in the health care system

- Health effects for staff and patients as a result of indoor air pollution, particularly among those who are environmentally sensitive

- Health effects—perhaps principally mental and social but also physical—resulting from the operation of landfills

Clearly, it is incumbent upon the health care system to reduce not only its environmental impact but also its health impact.

Reducing Health Care's Environmental and Health Impact

The hospital of the future should be the most environmentally friendly and healthy building in the community. Fortunately, there is a growing awareness of both the need for hospitals to be green, and practical examples of how this can be accomplished.

Energy Conservation

Recognizing the significant energy conservation potential in the health care sector, EPA administrator Christine Whitman launched an Energy Star energy performance rating tool for hospitals in November 2001. This performance benchmarking tool is free and confidential, allowing hospitals to compare their energy performance with that of other, similar facilities.

In the first year, only three of one hundred hospitals earned the Energy Star label by scoring over seventy-five on a nationwide scale of one to a hundred, based on data provided by the hospitals through EPA's Web-based energy efficiency pilot program.

Memorial Hospital of Carbondale, Illinois, one of the award recipients, has been undertaking energy efficiency improvements since 1979, including installing a central chilled water system, recovering heat from internal spaces for uses elsewhere in the hospital, and using a computerized energy management system. The hospital has also developed a vigilant engineering staff, aware of energy use and skilled in preventive maintenance in order to maximize energy efficiency while maintaining patient comfort.

As a result, total energy use at Memorial Hospital has increased only slightly since 1979, in spite of a doubling in size. Moreover, the hospital takes its efforts beyond its walls, being involved in a community-wide coalition to promote energy conservation in the community (Southern Illinois Healthcare News, 2001).

Canadian hospitals have also made strides in energy efficiency. Norfolk General Hospital in Ontario has decreased its overall energy budget by 22 percent, with a savings of at least $132,000 per year, every year since 1995. Among other things, it has replaced its three boilers and its cooling tower with smaller, more energy-efficient versions, it has used more efficient motors, fans, pumps, and lighting, and it has improved roof insulation and lowered the temperature of supply air in the winter and increased it in the summer, without adversely affecting staff and patient comfort levels.

Orillia Soldiers Memorial Hospital in Ontario, Canada, has operated a natural gas-powered cogeneration plant since 1991. The plant supplies 90 percent of the hospital's electrical power, while providing hot water and steam for the building. The hospital is now licensed to sell surplus power to the Ontario electric grid. The payback time for this plant was five to six years, and annual savings are over $200,000 (Canadian Coalition for Green Health Care, 2001).

Resource Conservation and Solid Waste Reduction

The core of solid waste reduction is to practice the "3Rs"—reduce, reuse, and recycle. Not only are there environmental and health benefits as a result of reducing waste, there are also economic benefits. For example, the average expenditure on waste management at Toronto's Hospital for Sick Children in the early 1990s approached $1.2 million, and the hospital had no recycling programs in place. As of 1998, the hospital had achieved the following in its drive to better handle its wastes:

- An 80 percent reduction in biomedical waste volume between 1992/3 and 2000/1, with these wastes falling from 4 percent of total wastes by volume to 1 percent

- A 78 percent increase in recycling over the same time period, rising from 6 percent of waste by volume to 47 percent

- A 6.7 percent reduction in the weight of materials going to landfill over the same period, falling from 90 percent of volume to 52 percent, despite filling 650,000 square feet of new space

- A reduction of annual waste management costs from $560,000 in 1992/3 to $107,097 in 2000/01 (Canadian Coalition for Green Health Care, 2001)

Pollution Prevention

Pollution prevention begins with avoiding, or at least reducing, the use of toxic substances. Given that the hospital is "home" to patients twenty-four hours a day, the sources of indoor air pollution need to be reduced, as do the emissions of toxic substances from the hospital to the wider environment.

It is particularly important that the health care system seek to reduce its use of toxic materials. One place to begin is with substances that are, by design, intended to harm living organisms. Given the growing scientific and public concern about the widespread use of pesticides, hospitals and other health care facilities should minimize their use of pesticides in their grounds and gardens. At the very least, an integrated pest management strategy should be employed. A number of Canadian hospitals have begun to take steps to reduce their use of toxic substances in recent years. For example, St. Mary's General Hospital in Kitchener, Ontario, winner of the 2001 Green Health Care Award in the Pollution Prevention category, has a "no chemical" lawn and grounds management policy. This policy includes the use of natural pest and weed control methods, microbiological methods of pest reduction, and a project to plan the grounds in line with this requirement.

Another class of toxic substances that is receiving growing attention is cleaning agents and disinfectants, some of which may have adverse effects on the environment or on the health of workers:

• Hackensack University Medical Center in New Jersey has developed a chemical cleaning product selection process that includes specifications (primarily relating to safety issues) that are absolutely required for product selection to proceed as well as criteria that are not essential but are important in product selection. These specifications and criteria cover individual, environmental, community, and public health concerns.

• Similarly, the Vienna Hospital Association has established criteria for environmentally friendly cleaning products. In their initial review of their use of cleaning products, they found that fifteen of forty-five products were heavily polluting the environment. Under their new purchasing criteria, of 175 products offered, only 20 were ecologically benign, 20 were ecologically acceptable, 105 were not acceptable, and 30 were acceptable but too expensive (Klausbruckner, 2001).

Useful resources for purchasing less toxic, green cleaners include the Janitorial Products Pollution Prevention Project (http://www.westp2net.org/janitorial/jp4.htm) and, in Canada, cleaning products that have been approved by the Canadian Environmental Choice Program (http://www.environmentalchoice.com/index_main.cfm).

In other cases, toxic materials such as laboratory chemicals, radioisotopes used in diagnosis and treatment, and cytotoxic drugs are so integral to the operation of the health care system that their use cannot be readily discontinued. The safe management and disposal of these substances is then a priority.

Creating Healthy Indoor Environments

One of the first responsibilities of a hospital must be to ensure that the physical environment of the hospital does not make patients, visitors, or staff members ill. Yet the combination of sealed buildings, synthetic materials, emissions from hospital and office equipment, and the use of multiple cleaning and disinfecting agents can all contribute to poor indoor air quality in hospitals, known as the "sick building syndrome." But good building design and management can overcome many of the problems that contribute to poor indoor air quality. This calls for paying attention to the materials used in the construction, the internal fittings, the equipment and furnishing of the building, and the ongoing operation, maintenance, and cleaning of the facility.

A Comprehensive Approach

It has become increasingly clear that if the environmental impact of health care is to be reduced, a comprehensive and long-term approach is needed that incorporates many strategies, including green building design, environmentally responsible purchasing, the adoption of environmental management systems, and the seeking of ISO 14001 accreditation (a voluntary standard put forward by the International Standards Organization in Geneva). This comprehensive approach is being adopted in part because hospitals are being required to meet tougher environmental standards for accreditation. The Canadian Council for Health Services Accreditation, for example, has strengthened its environmental standard in recent years. In addition, national and international coalitions have emerged in the United States, Canada, and elsewhere to promote and support the greening of health care.

Designing Green and Healthy Buildings

Environmentally friendly design has been a focus in the residential and commercial building sectors for many years. Clearly, this experience can be transferred to the design and construction of health care facilities.

One recent development that highlights the growing commitment to green or sustainable design in the health care sector is the launching in 2002 by the American Society for Health Care Engineering (in conjunction with the American Institute of Architects' Academy of Architecture for Health) of sustainable design awards (http://www.ashe.org). These awards are intended to recognize health care sector design projects in the area of green design and construction—in particular, with respect to

- Global climate change

- Toxics reduction

- Healthy indoor environments

- Stratospheric ozone layer protection

- Minimization and depletion of natural resources

- Reduction of energy and water consumption

There will be both a design award and a facility award, with the first awards to be given out in 2003 at the ASHE International Conference and Exhibition on Health Facility Planning, Design, and Construction.

At the same time, the ASHE's Green Building Committee has published a guidance statement on green health care construction. Noting that such an approach is consistent with the AHA's recent voluntary agreement with the EPA, the guidance statement suggests that green building design and construction can protect health on three levels:

1. Protecting the immediate health of building occupants (patients, staff members, and visitors), particularly through measures to ensure good indoor air quality, as well as access to daylight

2. Protecting the health of the surrounding community, particularly by reducing toxic emissions to water and air and through energy conservation and water management

3. Protecting the health of the larger global community and natural resources through reducing greenhouse gas emissions, avoiding the use and release of persistent organic pollutants, and preventing the release of substances that damage the stratospheric ozone layer

In March 2002, Kaiser Permanente adopted a position statement on green buildings, which reads as follows:

The mission of Kaiser Permanente (KP) is to improve the health of the communities we serve. In recognition of the critical linkages between environmental health and public health, it is KP's desire to limit adverse impacts upon the environment resulting from the siting, design, construction and operation of our health care facilities. We will address the life-cycle impacts of facilities through design and construction standards, selection of materials and equipment, and maintenance practices.

Additionally, KP will require architects, engineers and contractors to specify commercially available, cost-competitive materials, products, technologies and processes, where appropriate, that have a positive impact, or limit any negative impact on environmental quality and human health (Gerwig, 2002).

Green Purchasing

One of the important strategies for reducing environmental impact is to alter purchasing policies so as to purchase fewer environmentally harmful products. Several large group purchasing organizations (between them representing more than three-quarters of all U.S. hospitals) described their growing commitment to environmentally responsible purchasing. One group, Broadlane, reported that it had switched to PVC-free bags in 1996, whereas another, Consorta, reported switching to PVC- and DEHP-free enteric feeding tubes. And the largest, Premier, has on its Web site (http://www.premierinc.com/all/safety/resources/EPP/index.htm) a section on environmentally preferable purchasing.

In Massachusetts, the Office of Technical Assistance (OTA) of the Executive Office of Environmental Affairs offers a variety of special programs designed to meet the specific pollution prevention and compliance assistance needs of Massachusetts facilities. OTA is also a sponsor of the Healthcare Environmentally Preferable Purchasing (EPP) Network, a bimonthly forum for health care materials managers and other interested personnel to share information on environmental purchasing. Another very useful resource is the

Sustainable Hospitals Project in Lowell, Massachusetts, which has an on-line clearing house featuring a host of alternative green products (http://www.sustainablehospitals.org).

The Environmental Choice Program in Ottawa, Ontario (http://www.environmentalchoice.com), is Canada's only national and comprehensive eco-labeling program. Products and services certified by the Environmental Choice Program have proved to have less of an impact on the environment because of how they are manufactured, consumed, or disposed of. Certification of products and services is based on compliance with stringent environmental criteria that are established in consultation with industry, environmental groups, and independent experts and are based on research into the life cycle impacts of a product or service.

As the environmental and related health impacts of health care become more apparent, we can expect to see a growing movement toward environmentally responsible, green procurement, with respect not only to PVC but also to other potentially environmentally damaging and health-harmful products used in health care—from cleaners to pesticides, from IV bags to mercury-containing products, from disposable products to energy-inefficient equipment.

Environmental Management Systems and Standards

The greening of health care, as with the greening of any other large enterprise, is a complicated process. That is why groups that are engaged extensively in this issue stress the importance of adopting an environmental management strategy (EMS), which is also central to ISO 14001.

The adoption of an EMS requires commitment to environmental responsibility at the highest level—preferably expressed as part of the organization's core values and mission—to the implementation of a greening strategy, coupled with the creation of an interdepartmental "green team," or environmental management team, to manage the process. This team needs to be accountable to the executive team and needs to include members from all relevant departments, including service providers, housekeepers, and physical plant operators.

The adoption of an EMS and the creation of a green team are a key part of the environmental component of the new accreditation standard put forward by the Canadian Council for Health Services Accreditation. The council has included guidelines for environmental management in its standards since 1995. In order to be accredited, organizations are required to establish an environmental management team and manage the physical environment so as to ensure the safety of patients/clients and staff members.

Green Health Care Coalitions and Organizations

As the evidence on the environmental impact of health care becomes more widely discussed, a growing number of organizations have emerged in recent years to address these challenges. Among the most important are:

Health Care Without Harm. This U.S.-based coalition includes 347 organizations in thirty-seven countries in Africa, Asia, Central America, Europe, the Middle East, and North and South America. Health Care Without Harm's principal goals are to

- Eliminate the nonessential incineration of medical waste and to promote safe materials use and treatment practices

- Phase out the use of PVC plastics and persistent toxic chemicals in health care and to build momentum for a broader PVC phaseout campaign

- Phase out the use of mercury in all aspects of the health care industry

- Develop health-based standards for medical waste management and recognize and implement the public's right to know about chemical use in the health care industry

- Develop siting and transportation guidelines that conform to the principles of environmental justice and state that no communities should be poisoned by medical waste treatment and disposal

The coalition has a large number of publications and resource materials available at its Web site (http://www.noharm.org).

The Canadian Coalition for Green Health Care. This coalition was formed in 2000 by a group of national health care and environmental organizations as a result of a workshop convened by the Canadian Association of Physicians for the Environment, and it is funded in part by the U.S.-based Health Care Without Harm Coalition and Great Lakes United. The coalition is committed to encouraging the adoption of resource conservation and pollution prevention principles, as well as effective environmental management systems, without compromising safety and care, so as to protect human health and reduce the Canadian health care system's ecological impact. The booklet *Green Hospitals,* which provides a summary of the ten case studies and a detailed seventy-page report—"Doing Less Harm"—on assessing and reducing the environmental and health impact of Canada's health care system, is available at the coalition's Web site (http://www.greenhealthcare.ca).

Hospitals for a Healthy Environment (H2E) is a program that was created in 1998 by the AHA and the EPA. In 2001, the program was relaunched as a partnership between the EPA, the AHA, the American Nurses Association, and Health Care Without Harm to focus on

- Virtually eliminating mercury-containing waste from hospitals' waste streams by 2005

- Reducing the overall volume of waste (both regulated and nonregulated waste) by 33 percent by 2005 and by 50 percent by 2010

- Identifying hazardous substances for pollution prevention and waste reduction opportunities, including hazardous chemicals and persistent, bioaccumulative, and toxic pollutants

The H2E Web site (http://www.h2e-online.org) provides tools, resources, and case studies regarding these issues, as well as information on green purchasing and other technical resources. A list serve is also available for health care professionals to discuss technical information and practical strategies for pollution prevention. H2E has also established a number of recognition and award programs, including the H2E Environmental Leadership Award, which is given annually to facilities that have active, ongoing waste and mercury-use reduction programs and are setting the industry standard for environmental policies at other hospitals.

The Canadian Centre for Pollution Prevention (C2P2) encourages actions that avoid or minimize the creation of pollutants to foster a healthier environment and sustainable society. Serving as a catalyst for change, C2P2 disseminates information so that others include pollution prevention in their decision making. The centre has recently updated the Healthcare EnviroNet Web site (http://www.c2p2online.com), and it delivers a unique collection of Canadian-based information, including:

- Green alternatives for health care facilities

- Regulatory updates and government initiatives

- Canadian case studies

The *Sustainable Hospitals Project*, a project of The Lowell
Center for Sustainable Production at the University of
Massachusetts at Lowell, provides technical support to
the health care industry for selecting products and work
practices that eliminate or reduce occupational and environmental hazards, maintain quality patient care, and
contain costs. Key components of the project include
the Sustainable Hospitals Clearinghouse (http://www.
sustainablehospitals.org), with on-line information about
alternatives to products containing mercury, latex, PVC,
and other potentially harmful materials. The site includes
alternative product lists and vendor information, as well
as key user considerations for the products.

The Green Hospital of the Future

Looking to the future, what would a green hospital be like? Here
are some suggestions:

- A green hospital would be designed to make the best use
  of passive solar energy by being oriented to the sun and
  sheltered from northerly winds, as well as using natural
  shade and ventilation for cooling in the summer.

- A green hospital would use solar, wind, and other
  renewable forms of energy, as well as environmentally
  friendly fuel cells, and it would also use cogeneration
  technologies to use energy with maximum efficiency.

- The green hospital's wastes would be minimized by
  reducing unnecessary use of resources, using reusable
  materials wherever possible in place of disposables, and
  recycling paper, plastics, metals, and other materials.

- At a green hospital, all waste disposal would use the least
  polluting option available and would meet the highest

standards for the protection of human and ecosystem health, with composting of organic wastes whenever possible.

The green hospital would avoid the use of toxic materials as much as possible, using green purchasing cooperatives to leverage the production of alternative environmentally friendly products, using green cleaners, integrated pest management, and other clean products and technologies.

The green hospital would use low-emission, nontoxic materials in its construction and in all aspects of its operation, ensuring a high level of indoor air quality. The hospital might even use "breathing wall" technology to provide both air purification and an attractive indoor natural ecosystem. It would use "living machine" sewage treatment technologies to treat its wastes on site.

In short, the hospital of the future, and especially the Planetree hospital of the future, can and should be the most environmentally friendly and healthiest building in the community, minimizing the harm it does to the environment and the health of the many species, including humans, who live in it.

Note

1. Among the issues identified in this report is the need for energy conservation to be designed into buildings and for health care facilities to be sited so that public transport, biking, and walking are possible and car use is reduced. The report is available at http://www.kingsfund.org.uk.

References

Canadian Centre for Pollution Prevention and Broadhurst Environmental Management, Inc. *Health Care Pollution Prevention and Environmental Management Resource Guide*. Sarnia: Canadian Centre for Pollution Prevention, 1996.

Canadian Coalition for Green Health Care. "Green Hospitals: Success Stories of Environmentally Responsible Health Care." 2001. [Available as a downloadable PDF file in the Resources section at www.greenhealthcare.ca].

Centers for Medicare and Medicaid Services. "Table 1: National Health
    Expenditures and Selected Economic Indicators, Levels and Average
    Annual Percent Change: Selected Calendar Years 1980–2011."
    [http://cms.hhs.gov/statistics/nhe/projections-2001/highlights.asp]. 2002.
Centre for the Analysis and Dissemination of Demonstrated Energy Technolo-
    gies. *Saving Energy with Energy Efficiency in Hospitals*. Sittard, The Nether-
    lands: Centre for the Analysis and Dissemination of Demonstrated Energy
    Technologies, 1997. [http://www.caddet-ee.org/brochures/display.php?id=1091].
Daughton, C., and Ternes, T. "Pharmaceuticals and Personal Care Products in
    the Environment: Agents of Subtle Change?" *Environmental Health Per-
    spectives*, 1999, *107* (supp. 6), 907–936.
Environment Canada, Ontario Region. Fact sheet: "Mercury Reduction in the
    Health Care Sector." N. d.
Germain, S. "The Ecological Footprint of Lion's Gate Hospital." *Hospital Quar-
    terly*, 2002, 5(2), 61–66.
Gerwig, K. "Position Statement on Green Buildings." National Resource Con-
    servation and National Environmental Health and Safety Operations,
    Kaiser Permanente, Oakland, Calif., Mar. 2002.
Green Design Initiative. "Economic Input-Output Life Cycle Assessment."
    Carnegie Mellon University. [http://www.eiolca.net]. 2000.
Hancock, T., and Davies, K. "The Health Implications of Global Change:
    A Canadian Perspective." A paper for the Rio +5 Forum, prepared for Envi-
    ronment Canada under the auspices of the Royal Society of Canada's Cana-
    dian Global Change Program. Ottawa: The Royal Society of Canada, 1997.
Hawken, P., Lovins, A., and Lovins, L. H. *Natural Capitalism: Creating the Next
    Industrial Revolution*. Boston: Little, Brown, 1999.
Health Care Without Harm. *Green Hospitals*, 1998. [Also available at
    http://www.noharm.org].
Health Care Without Harm. Fact Sheet: "Dioxin, PVC, and Health Care
    Institutions." Falls Church, Va.: Health Care Without Harm, 2001.
Health Care Without Harm. "DEHP Exposures During the Medical Care of Infants."
    Publication 3-6 of *Going Green: A Resource Kit for Pollution Prevention in
    Health Care*. Falls Church, Va.: Health Care Without Harm, 2002.
Henschel, K. P., Wenzel, A., Diedrich, M., and Fliedner, A. "Environmental
    Hazard Assessment of Pharmaceuticals." *Regulatory Toxicology and Pharma-
    cology*, 1997, 25(3), 220–225.
Homer, J. "Adverse Health Effect of Toxic Chemicals in the Work Environ-
    ment." A presentation at the CleanMed 2001 Conference, Boston,
    Mass., 2001.

Intergovernmental Panel on Climate Change. *Climate Change 1995: The Second Assessment Report, Volume 2.* Cambridge, Mass.: Cambridge University Press, 1996.

Klausbruckner, B. "The Vienna Hospital Association's Environmental Policies and Programs." A presentation at the CleanMed 2001 Conference, Boston, Mass., 2001.

McCarthy, J. and others, Intergovernmental Panel on Climate Change. "Climate Change 2001: Impacts, Adaptation and Vulnerability." Cambridge, England: Cambridge University Press, 2001.

McMichael, A. J., and others. *Climate Change and Human Health.* Geneva: World Health Organization, 1996.

Natural Resources Canada. *Energy in Canada 2000.* Ottawa: Natural Resources Canada, 2000.

Ontario Medical Association. *Illness Costs of Air Pollution.* Toronto: Ontario Medical Association, 2000.

Romm, J., and Ervin, C. "How Energy Policies Affect Public Health." *Public Health Reports,* 1996, *111*(5), 390–399.

Southern Illinois Healthcare News. [http://www.sih.net/newswire.nsf/main]. Dec. 21, 2001.

Tieszen, M., and Gruenberg, J. "A Quantitative, Qualitative and Critical Assessment of Surgical Waste." *JAMA,* 1992, *267*(20), 2765–2768.

U.S. Department of Energy, Energy Information Administration. "A Look at Commercial Buildings in 1995: Characteristics, Energy Consumption, and Energy Expenditures." Washington, D.C.: U.S. Department of Energy, 2002.

Wackernagel, M., and Rees, W. E. *Our Ecological Footprint: Reducing Human Impact on the Earth.* Gabriola Island, B.C.; Philadelphia, Pa.: New Society Publishers, 1996.

Weinhold, B. "Making Health Care Healthier: A Prescription for Change." *Environmental Health Perspectives,* 2001, *109*(8), A370–A377.

Whitman, C. Quoted on EPA Web site [http://www.epa.gov/epahome/headline2_111601.htm)]. Nov. 16, 2001.

World Resources Institute. *World Resources 1998–99: Health and Environment.* New York: Oxford University Press, 1998.

14

Adapting Patient-Centered Care to the Long-Term Care Environment

Allan Komarek

To create a healing environment in a long-term care environment, four cornerstones of any health care model must be considered: physical care, socialization, psychological care, and consideration of spiritual needs. Yet this is not enough. It is the attitude of the people delivering that care that creates a healing environment. Walk into the most elegantly appointed hotel in the world and you will see the extrinsic; talk to the person at the front desk and you will feel the intrinsic. It is the human interaction that makes us feel special or, conversely, objectifies us.

The attitude of the caregivers in a long-term care environment must match the beauty of the surroundings, and attitudes cannot be legislated. It is the intrinsic factor that differentiates the Planetree long-term care environment. The walls can be covered with beautiful artwork, harps can play in the entry, and activities can be tailored to meet the psychosocial needs of the resident, and the resident will always be able to tell what is in the hearts of the caregivers.

Many of today's nursing homes have ostensibly created Planetree settings. The surroundings are homelike, the atmosphere is quiet, and the resident's rooms are filled with personal memorabilia. The interior design is often warm and beautiful, containing artwork and beautifully contrasting floor and wall coverings. Residents are dressed in their own clothing and are up in wheelchairs, pushing walkers, or sitting in lounges designed to encourage socialization.

They may be attending a rousing game of bingo, watching their favorite soap opera, or just sitting in a wheelchair watching the nurses as they go about their daily work. The dining room is beautifully appointed and the residents are urged to eat their meals in the company of other residents.

According to Mary Smith, director of the Overlook Center at Fauquier Hospital in Warrenton, Virginia, "long-term care facilities are far ahead of hospitals in customer-centered programs. We have always allowed family members to come and go, and the resident can bring anything from home because it is their home." Unfortunately, this has not always been the case.

Definition of Long-Term Care

Long-term care is a continuum of care that ranges from independent living facilities for the elderly to skilled care in a nursing facility for high-acuity patients. At the beginning of this continuum are retirement communities and assisted living facilities. In the middle of the continuum are board and care facilities and nursing facilities and at the end of the continuum are skilled nursing facilities that include rehabilitation services and specialized facilities such as Alzheimer's units. Typically, long-term care is associated with nursing care for clients unable to care for themselves.

Nursing homes (often called convalescent hospitals) offer two kinds of care. The first is the basic care that is required to maintain a resident's activities of daily living, which includes personal care, ambulation, supervision, and safety. The second is the skilled care that requires the services of a registered nurse for treatments and procedures on a regular basis. Skilled care also includes services provided by specially trained professionals, such as physical, occupational, and respiratory therapists.

The services offered in nursing homes include room and board, the monitoring of medication, personal care, and access to emergency care and social and recreational activities. Regulations require that patients have their own unique care plan, which must be comprehensive.

Medicaid is the primary payment mechanism for most nursing home stays. It is a common misconception that Medicare covers the cost of nursing home care. In fact, the Medicare benefit only covers the first hundred days of care in a skilled nursing facility. This kind of care is often called "subacute" care. There is usually a heavy emphasis on rehabilitation during this time period. Private long-term care insurance is available to supplement Medicare. There are many long-term care insurance plans available and their terms vary from company to company.

Nursing homes have long been the focus of long-term care. One of the results of Medicare's change to prospective payment in the late 1970s and early 1980s was the acute care hospital's addition of long-term care beds. There was an economic incentive to move patients from acute care beds to long-term care beds. Before prospective payments, known as DRGs (diagnosis-related groupings), Medicare paid hospitals, based on what it cost the hospital to deliver care, which incentivized hospitals to keep patients in the acute care bed for as long as possible. With the advent of prospective payment, which paid hospitals a certain sum of money based on the patient's illness, hospitals were incentivized to move patients from the acute care setting as soon as possible. Nursing homes were unable to care for these sicker patients and there were not enough nursing home beds. Hospitals saw this as a way of saving money and increasing revenues and moved quickly to fill the gap.

Abuses

According to Paul Takahashi (1998), from the Mayo Clinic and Mayo Foundation in Rochester, Minnesota, "there is no greater challenge to health care providers than institutional mistreatment in long-term care." Takahashi gives examples of actual cases of abuse in long-term care:

- A patient's bedside commode is filled with urine and feces and ignored by the staff, despite a family request to empty it.

- A nursing home resident without pants on is in a wheelchair placed in the dining room, because the resident refused to get dressed.

- A long-term nursing home resident is a lifetime smoker but is forbidden to smoke under the new owner's no-smoking policy.

- A bed-bound nursing home resident has end-stage dementia, and a staff member finds another demented resident smothering her with a pillow.

- A husband and wife in a nursing home live in separate rooms, and a nursing assistant sees the husband strike his wife.

- A nursing home resident is found two blocks from the home, attempting to drown herself in a lake.

- A nursing home resident has a percutaneous endoscopic gastrostomy (PEG), and a staff member has to use wrist restraints to prevent the patient from pulling out the PEG tube.

- Three female nursing home residents with dementia have all developed—within two weeks—herpes in the pubic or buttocks area.

This list shows that defining abuse is difficult. It is also nearly impossible to uncover in many circumstances. Abuse includes physical abuse or neglect, psychological abuse or neglect, financial or material abuse, and violation of personal rights.

A "warehouse for the elderly" has long been the view of nursing homes. This view of long-term care includes images of forcing grandmother out of her home and into a cold, dark room staffed by incompetent and uncaring caregivers. Stories of long-term care facilities keeping the elderly in bed, causing bedsores, restraining them for no reason, dropping them—causing deadly fractures—and even physically and mentally abusing them abound. Consumer groups like the Citizens for Quality Nursing Home Care in Louisiana and the California Advocates for Nursing Home Reform are outgrowths of early abuses. These groups lobby their state and federal legislators for better protections for residents and have been successful in many areas.

Congress created tougher national long-term standards in 1987. These standards were attached to the Omnibus Budget Reconciliation Act and are now known as the OBRA standards. Based on provisions of the Omnibus Budget Reconciliation Act of 1987, the Health Care Finance Administration (HCFA) revised Medicare and Medicaid compliance requirements for long-term care facilities. The HCFA, now known as the Centers for Medicare and Medicaid Services, contracts with state agents, either public or private, to interpret OBRA regulations and implement site surveys.

In response, nursing homes created homelike atmospheres, though the care delivered was often anything but homelike. The literature is rife with articles that question the quality of care in nursing homes ("Nursing Home Rehabilitation Stay Proves Terminal," 1999; "Elderly Patient Repeatedly Injured in Nursing Home 'Accidents,'" 1999).

States such as California have long had regulations governing resident rights. In response to nursing home abuses, Medicare wrote a list of resident rights.

Rights of Nursing Home Residents

Following are the rights of nursing home residents:

- Nursing home residents have the right to see family members, ombudspersons, or other resident advocates,

physicians, service providers, and representatives of the
state and federal government.

- Residents may keep and use their personal possessions
  and clothing unless doing so would endanger health
  and safety.

- Residents have the right to apply for and receive
  Medicare and Medicaid benefits and cannot be asked
  to leave a home because they receive such benefits.

- A nursing home must treat all individuals the same,
  regardless of whether they are private payers or
  Medicare or Medicaid recipients.

- Residents have the right to keep their clinical and personal records confidential.

- Residents are entitled to lists of what services are paid
  by Medicare and Medicaid and the additional services
  for which the residents will be charged, plus the fees for
  those services.

- Residents have the right to choose their own personal
  physician.

- Residents have the right to be fully informed about
  their medical care.

- Residents have the right to participate in the planning
  of their care and treatment.

- Residents have the right to refuse treatment.

- Residents have the right to be free from mental and
  physical abuse.

- Residents cannot be kept apart from other residents
  against their will.

- Residents cannot be tied down or given drugs to restrain them if restraint is not necessary to treat their medical symptoms.

- Residents have the right to raise grievances and have them resolved quickly.

- Residents may participate in social, religious, and community activities to the extent that they do not interfere with the rights of other residents.

- Residents cannot be required to deposit their personal funds with the nursing home, and if they request that the home manage their funds, the home must do so according to state and federal record-keeping requirements.

- Residents have the right to privacy, including in their rooms, medical treatment, communications, visits, and meetings with family and resident groups.

- Residents have the right to review their medical records within twenty-four hours of making a request.

- Residents have the right to review the most recent state inspection report relating to the home.

- Residents must be given notice before their room or roommate is changed, and residents can refuse the transfer if the purpose is to move them from a Medicare bed to a Medicaid bed or vice versa.

- Residents have the right to stay in the nursing home and can only be removed if it is necessary for the resident's welfare, the resident no longer needs the facility's services, it is necessary to prevent harm to the health or safety of others in the facility, the resident fails to pay after reasonable notice, or the facility ceases to operate.

- Residents and their representatives have the right to thirty days' notice of a proposed transfer or discharge, and they have the right to appeal.

- Before transferring residents for hospitalization or therapy, the nursing home must inform them of the length of time that their beds will be held open for their return, called the "bedhold period."

- Residents returning from a hospital or therapeutic leave after expiration of the bedhold period have the right to be readmitted as soon as the first semi-private bed becomes available.

- Residents must be informed of their rights upon admission and must be given their rights in writing if so requested (Consumer Law Center, n.d.).

Building a Long-Term Care Healing Environment

Many of today's nursing homes have all the amenities. Rooms are decorated with the resident's personal belongings. Pictures of family members are hung on the walls, hallways have art hanging, and living rooms are beautifully appointed. Residents are dressed each morning and are asked to go to the dining room to take their meals. Their nutritional level has been assessed and their weight is monitored to ensure adequate nutrition. Intake and output is monitored to ensure adequate hydration and elimination. The resident sits at a table and is brought his or her exclusive diet as ordered by the physician. The staff is available to monitor and ensure that the resident is eating. Activities are provided, based on an assessment by an activities director, or even a recreation therapist. Physical care is attended to by registered nurses, licensed practical nurses, and nursing assistants. Some nursing homes even provide geriatricians and clinical nurse specialists. Social workers help the residents with problems they may have, whether financial or spiritual.

The nursing home environment has strived to be as homelike as possible. Regulations such as OBRA have attempted to legislate care. A superficial caring environment is often the result of these regulations. No legislative body has ever, or will ever, be able to regulate human attitudes. This is the Planetree difference.

Elements of the Planetree Model in Long-Term Care

Although the Planetree model was developed initially for acute care patients, it is equally as appropriate—and needed—in long-term care settings. With modest adjustments, the components of the model are easily adapted to a variety of health care environments.

Human Interactions

The healing environment in any long-term care setting must begin with respect for the resident and his or her uniqueness. The long-term care patient often feels a lack of respect, value, and dignity by the mere act of being placed in a nursing home. These feelings, along with others associated with aging, create a challenge for the staff of the long-term care unit.

It is not only the long-term care patient who is left with negative feelings. Often, the family is plagued with guilt for not being able to take care of the family member in the home. Fowler (1999) states, "Adult children may feel guilty as caregivers of parents because of beliefs valued throughout life," including:

- It is selfish to put my own needs ahead of those of others.

- No one can care for my parent as well as I.

- I must do it all and make everyone happy.

Add the guilt felt by adult children when admitting their aged parent to a nursing home and the feelings become almost unbearable. According to the organization Friends and Relatives of

Institutionalized Aged (1998–1999), "when families must place someone they love in a nursing home, they often feel guilty for not abiding by the tradition, failure because they could not continue to provide care and fear that others in their family and community will be critical without understanding the circumstances." These feelings of guilt, failure, and fear can be turned into feelings of participation, involvement, and usefulness through the care partner program.

Family Involvement

The Planetree Care Partner Program (described in Chapter Three) is at the crux of a successful transition into the nursing home environment for both the patient and the family. The staff can play a key role in assisting both the patient and the family in decreasing these negative feelings. The sensitivity of the staff to the presence of possible guilt feelings on the part of the family is the key to helping to diffuse the feeling. According to Friends and Relatives of Institutionalized Aged (1998–1999), "there are many ways to stay involved once a relative enters a nursing home. The family may even have more time and energy to provide love and support when they are not overwhelmed with providing daily health care." The staff can help the family member stay involved through the care partner program and can assist in supporting the patient, who is going through feelings of loss of dignity and respect.

Mark Clarfield (1998) lists the reduction of jargonesque fluency and "medicalese" as one of the main criteria for respect shown to the resident. He continues: "Not only do older patients require that their physician speak to them in plain English, but, for those who can understand it, speak to them with obvious respect. For example, unless patients direct you to do so, never call them by their first names." Unfortunately, words like "dear" and "honey" are used as terms of endearment and are perceived by the resident as indicating a lack of respect. Other forms of respect include knocking at the patient's door, introducing oneself, and listening to what the resident has to say.

Spirituality

Spirituality is an elusive aspect of long-term care. According to Sister Jean Roche (1997), "spirituality is better defined as that which fosters connectedness with creation, oneself, others, or God. . . . If a spiritual climate is to be created and maintained in any of the long-term care settings, the leadership must be attentive to the soul and spirit of the organization, providing opportunities that help staff members be aware of their own spiritual power." Many nursing homes invite ministers, rabbis, and other spiritual leaders to provide services for the residents, but it is the staff members who must continue to create an environment in which each resident feels that connectedness that Roche describes.

One of the ways in which organizations can assist employees in creating an environment that invites the connectedness desired by the resident is through an emphasis on values. Organizational values can define the culture leadership wishes to be created. What is important for long-term care employees is that they understand those values and how they can use them in their daily work. Values help the employees in their daily decision-making and in creating a spiritual atmosphere in which residents can thrive.

Creating a culture in which everyone learns to listen is important to the mental health of the resident. Even the aged need opportunities for soul searching. Providing opportunities for residents to heal the wounds in their lives due to death, losses, betrayals, or rejections creates a culture of connectedness. Residents and their family members need to be heard in order to feel supported. The people who are there to hear them are most often the nursing assistants and housekeepers.

One of the basic building blocks of Planetree is the staff retreat. It is through this retreat that the basic principles of respect and the creation of an environment of connectedness are reinforced with staff. It is through these retreats that staff members are reminded that the long-term resident is a human being with needs that should be recognized and honored. Warren Memorial Hospital in Front Royal, Virginia, devotes a special segment in its Planetree University staff development program that concentrates on dementia patients and the ways employees can help to normalize their lives.

Giving the health care consumer choice, and therefore, control, is a basic tenet in the Planetree environment. In long-term care, its relevance is even more evident. "One day, at a nursing home in Connecticut, elderly residents were each given a choice of house plants to care for and were asked to make a number of small decisions about their daily routines. A year and a half later, not only were these people more cheerful, active, and alert than a similar group in the same institution who were not given these choices and responsibilities, but many more of them were still alive. In fact, less than half as many of the decision-making, plant-minding residents had died as had those in the other group" (Langer, 1989).

The Ten Principles of the Eden Alternative

The Eden Alternative is a philosophy of care that was begun in a nursing home in upstate New York by founder Bill Thomas (2002) and his wife, Judy. They call it "a holistic environment." It is based on the following ten principles:

1. The three plagues of loneliness, helplessness, and boredom account for the bulk of suffering among Elders.

2. Life in an Elder-centered community revolves around close and continuing contact with children, plants, and animals. These ancient relationships provide young and old alike with a pathway to a life worth living.

3. Companionship is the antidote to loneliness. In an Elder-centered community we must provide easy access to human and animal companionship.

4. A healthy Elder-centered community seeks to balance the care that is being given, with the care that is being received.

Elders need opportunities to give care and caregivers need opportunities to receive care.

5. Variety and Spontaneity are the antidotes to boredom. The Elder-centered community is rich in opportunities to sample these ancient pleasures.

6. An Elder-centered community understands that passive entertainment cannot fill a human life.

7. The Elder-centered community takes medical treatment down from its pedestal and places it into the service of genuine human caring.

8. In an Elder-centered community, decisions should be made by the Elders or those as close to the Elders as possible.

9. An Elder-centered community understands human growth cannot be separated from human life.

10. Wise leadership is the lifeblood of any struggle against the Three Plagues. For it, there can be no substitute.

Thomas (2002) made rounds in this nursing home and found it lacking in humanity. He took over as administrator and the "Eden Alternative" was born. One of the wisdoms found by Thomas and his wife was that people need to give care as well as receive care to feel valuable. As Susan C. Eaton, assistant professor of public policy at the Wiener Center for Social Policy for the John F. Kennedy School of Government at Harvard University, states, "The Eden paradigm allowed elders to care for animals, birds, and children as well as each other."

Arts and Activities

The cornerstone of any nursing home is the activities program, which often becomes the Planetree healing arts program. The activities program provides the nutrition for the soul. It is through these programs that many of the resident's psychosocial, physical, and spiritual needs are met. Typically, the goals of activity programs are

- Socialization daily out of the room to prevent boredom and homesickness and to have a more meaningful environment

- Reorientation to self, time, date, and activities of daily living

- Self-expression and communication through the arts including, but not limited to, cooking, dancing (movement), singing, and painting

- Building self-esteem

Typical activities include

- Birthday parties, special occasion parties, holiday parties, farewell parties

- Religious services

- Card and board games

- Cooking classes

- Special visitations

- Arts and crafts

- Entertainment from all categories

- Exercise/movement/dance

- Bingo

- Aroma therapy

- Reading to residents

- Grooming activities (haircuts, makeup)

- Resident councils

- Outings

- Pet therapy

- Movie/television/music

Through these activities, the goal of the staff is to have each resident spend more than thirty minutes outside of his or her room on a daily basis. A feeling of isolation resulting from placement in a nursing home can lead the resident toward depression. These activities are designed to encourage socialization and a feeling of belonging. Each of the residents has left his or her own home and his or her own "society" and must assimilate into this new society. As the resident becomes more socialized to the surroundings, the goals change to include increasing his or her self-esteem. As self-esteem increases, so does the level of participation in activities. The benefits become self-evident.

Libraries on the unit provide reading material for enjoyment and education for the resident. Warren Memorial has a library for its residents who enjoy reading. Books with large print or books on tape are especially popular and provide relief from boredom.

It is through the activity program that care partners can become a reality in the long-term care environment. Schools now often require community service as a prerequisite for graduation, and combining this with the needs of a resident can, and does, produce magic. Someone from the resident's family is the ideal care partner. His or her involvement in the care, from admission to discharge, will help both the resident and the family in many ways.

Residents who are bed-bound can also benefit from bedside activities programs such as books on tape, television, radio, sensory stimulation (including touch, smell, taste, and auditory), volunteer/family visits, and orientation to family and self through the use of pictures and date and time. The long-term care unit at Delano Regional Medical Center in Delano, California, has many comatose patients. Those patients are included in the activities program through the use of volunteer readers. Televisions are tuned into the residents' favorite programs and the kind of music preferred by the comatose resident is played on the radio. When patients are first admitted, special care is taken to interview the family about the resident's likes and dislikes in television and radio programming. Favorite authors and books are also discussed. Staff members talk to the residents as if they are hearing every word, and staff are encouraged to comment on family pictures in the room.

The long-term goals of activity programs include the following:

• The resident will comfortably socialize with others.

• The resident will participate actively in activities without encouragement.

• The resident will make friends in the facility.

• The resident will maintain personal dignity.

Of course, the final goal is to discharge the resident home. But often, the resident achieves socialization at a higher level in a nursing facility than at home. When the resident is discharged, it is incumbent upon the social workers to find support for the resident that equals or exceeds the activity level the resident found in the nursing facility.

Pet Therapy

The use of animals as therapy in long-term care is now recognized as part of the healing process. It is well documented that dogs have a calming and therapeutic effect and can help people cope with emotional issues. They offer physical contact and, according to Steve Reiman (2000), "for long-term care residents, it is not so much the stress of daily problems, but the boredom, loneliness, and lack of control." Reiman continues: "Dogs offer themselves to patients with joy, unconditional love, great affection, and unending patience. They can have a profound ability to touch residents not engaged by other kinds of therapies. While it may be difficult to quantify the benefits of dog therapy with hard scientific evidence, the magical interaction possible between animal and human is unmistakable. Tears dry, frowns transform into smiles, inactive hands caress soft fur. Silence becomes a conversation of whispers in a dog's ear."

Aroma Therapy

Aroma therapy can be used in the long-term care environment to help patients recall pleasant memories, and it opens the lines of communication between residents and between residents and staff members. Aromas from the kitchen can stimulate the appetite and may be an aid to good nutrition.

Architectural Design

Architectural design in the long-term care environment must be conducive to health and healing. Design usually takes the needs of the staff into consideration but rarely the needs of the residents. Phyllis Stoneburner, vice president for patient care services at Warren Memorial Hospital, has created an environment where there are no straight hallways. All corridors are shortened so that pods, or communities of eight, are created. There is a place for sitting within the pods to encourage socialization as well as intimate family spaces. As you twist and turn through the corridors, you are greeted by little surprises such as a fish tank, a garden, a music room, a "guys" room, and a library. You also find a two-story aviary and bold colors like gold, burgundy, green, and teal—non–nursing home colors. The effect is one of delight in discovery. Design defeats boredom.

Warren Memorial has given great thought to the environment for Alzheimer's patients. The unit is on the garden level (a pseudonym for the first floor). There are wander gardens so that the resident can go in and out freely. The resident also sees a basketball hoop, an old car in which he or she can pretend to travel, a clothesline, water gardens, and pockets of activity. There are also multigenerational activities for children.

Ann Saczuk, the geriatrics and extended care line manager at the Veterans Administration Hospital in Batavia, New York, has a dream of a Dementia Life Center, where patients would never have to be told no by the staff. "There would be nothing off limits. There would be food when they were hungry, activity when they wanted, sleep when they wanted, exercise to burn off anxiety, music to calm, therapies to soothe, fresh air any season, a pet to bond with, and family involvement. Staff would recognize that this is the patients' home and that they are just 'visiting' for their eight-hour shift" (interview, March 2002). Saczuk's vision for the Dementia Life Center includes the following ideas:

Entry

- Create a pseudo house entry; use actual home-type door, siding, lighting, and awning

- Resident artist to create landscaping around entry, including a sycamore tree, whose branches would extend over the ceiling of the entry

- Place a brass plate on the door, saying "Life Center"

Entry Hallway

- Install carpet, textured wall paper, and wall sconces that provide soft lighting

- Wall-paper the back side of the entry door, to blend in and reduce noticeableness by patients as they exit

- Include a lighted drinking fountain alcove

Former Nurses' Station

- Convert to quiet alcove by installing lattice work from counter to ceiling and using artificial vine plants to cover

- Furnish soft couches and chairs

- Install soft lighting

- Include a water feature in the corner

- Provide music

Therapy Tub Room

- Use the new Apollo tub as a therapy device

- Supply bath oils and aroma therapy (lavender especially) for the water

- Provide scented candles

- Include aftershave products

- Supply large towels and a towel warmer

- Provide music

Alternative Therapy Room

- Include a massage table for use by the chiropractor, massage therapist, and Reiki therapist

- Offer massage services to family members as well as to patients

- Include handheld massage devices for staff use

- Add an old-fashioned scalp vibrator that barbers used to use after cutting hair

Guest Room

- Create hotel-like rooms (with adjoining bathrooms) for family members to stay overnight in if they wish; such rooms may be used for conjugal visits

- Include a quiet room

- Include a female patient room (Veterans Administration facilities have a majority of male patients)

Solarium

- Engage a resident artist to paint a garden with small animals on the walls

- Include a resident pet room

- Provide outdoor furniture

- Provide stuffed animals for residents to hold

Multisensory Room

- Provide structured but independent activity for patients

- Provide diversional opportunities that include musical instruments and a wide range of very interesting objects to touch, feel, throw, cuddle, look at, listen to, and take apart

- Provide a lava lamp and projector for light images on the ceiling

- Provide a recliner chair with massage and heat

- Supply and stock a fish tank

Military Room

- Create a wall of honor for pictures of current and past residents in uniform

- Include pictures of military equipment, vehicles, planes, and so on

- Supply military memorabilia to handle—such as fatigues, helmets, boots, toy tanks, badges, and ribbons

- Supply military music

- Include a tent-like structure in one corner

- Include flags

Music Room

- Install a stereo system with music from the thirties, forties, and fifties

- Create a dance floor

- Supply posters from the movies or big bands

Art Room

- Have one long wall that can be painted on and then wiped down, to allow patients to "paint the house"

- Provide easels and art materials

- Provide clay

- Invite art students from a local college

Laundry Room

- Install a washer and dryer

- Use the laundry room for "work assignments" of folding towels and clothes

- Allow families to wash patient clothing while they are visiting

Fitness Room

- Supply exercise mats and appropriate equipment

- Provide music

Family Resource Center

- Include a quiet room that is away from activities

- Provide computers that have Internet access

- Create a library that is well stocked with health care materials and other types of literature

- Include a counseling room

Outside Area

- Create a fenced-in yard with a gazebo

- Create a walking pathway

- Provide an adult sandbox

- Include a smoking area

- Provide a swing and a rocker

- Create a garden for flowers and vegetables

- Include a horse shoe pit

Saczuk continues: "This type of unique facility would attract students from local colleges and universities to do clinical rotations with us, especially in psychology, social work, recreation and occupational therapies, music therapy, art therapy, nursing, [and] dietetics, advancing the field of caring for these often overlooked patients" (interview, March 2002).

Ten Kerselaere

In Belgium, the Catholic Health Insurance Company, working in collaboration with a team of medical and nursing advisers, created a geriatric center called Ten Kerselaere (the Cherry Orchard). Franz Baro and R. Dom, of the Department of Brain and Behavior Research at the University of Leuven, Belgium, state, "In contrast (to acute care) long-term care facilities should offer a caring medical attendance, a devoted, well-trained paramedical and nursing staff, a well-organized and appealing hotel service, a peaceful and home-like atmosphere with respect for privacy and territory, as well as a stimulating environment and recreational possibilities."

According to Baro and Dom (n.d.),

> to realize these objectives and this philosophy, the architect designed Ten Kerselaere to resemble a small, dynamic village where all normal daily activities take place. Rather than long narrow corridors, there are wide streets, squares, and street corners, a cafe, beauty parlor, chapel, shops, exhibits, and happenings, attracting residents to a more social life style. Strolls are encouraged via sensory stimulation in the form of children's playgrounds, small livestock, birds, flowers, greenery. Therapeutic and rehabilitation activities are discretely open

for all to see, avoiding apprehension and suspicion about the unknown among the residents. Integrated into daily living, they give a positive view of their potential bene-fits to residents, family, and visitors alike.

Baro and Dom add that ultimately, the residents of Ten Kerse-laere live in an environment that "blends activities and services and creates a harmonious atmosphere."

Nutritional and Nurturing Aspects of Food

Many residents of long-term care facilities are at risk for nutritional deficiencies. A recent study (Kamel, Karcic, Karcic, and Barghouthi, 2000) concluded that "elderly patients admitted from a nursing home to a hospital have significantly worse markers of nutritional status, compared with elderly patients admitted from the commu-nity." The study went on to point out that "this difference is mainly attributed to increased comorbidity, polypharmacy, and increased dependency in the activities of daily living among patients admitted from a nursing home. Careful attention should be paid to the nutritional status of this nutritionally high-risk group of patients."

According to Dennis Sullivan (2000), "clinically, undernutri-tion manifests as an increased susceptibility to infection, delayed wound healing, reduced rates of drug metabolism, and impairment of both physical and cognitive function."

Depression and dementia are often the cause of weight loss. One study found that depression is present in 8 to 38 percent of residents and that treatment has been shown to result in the regaining of lost weight. Demented patients often forget to eat (Fitten, Morley, and Gross, 1989; Kahn, 1995; Morley, 1996). Depression falls into the category of appetite suppressants, whereas dementia falls into the category of barriers to eating. Other appetite suppressants include medication, the environment, subclinical infections, gastrointesti-nal disorders, metabolic disorders, overly restrictive diets, and cultural considerations. Barriers to eating include lack of feeding assistance, poor oral and dental status, nonoptimal food consistency, and rigid meal policies.

Eliminating the appetite suppressants and barriers to eating are the Planetree challenge in long-term care. Management of undernutrition entails early detection and management of treatable disorders. Diagnosing and treating depression are an important first step. Other treatments include:

- Eliminating anorexigenic drugs

- Eliminating unnecessary dietary restrictions

- Creating an environment conducive to eating

- Providing assistance with feeding, especially of residents with dementia

- Responding to ethnic food preferences

- Involving residents in menu revision and food selection

To help prevent weight loss in residents with dementia, the Bishop Wicke Health and Care Center in Shelton, Connecticut, created a "finger foods" program for those unable to eat using utensils. To help residents maintain their independence and dignity by being able to feed themselves, each meal includes at least two food items that can be picked up with the fingers, such as sandwiches, hamburgers, hot dogs, carrot sticks, apples, or cookies. According to Moira Ethier, rehabilitation coordinator, the residents on the "finger food" program have stopped losing weight, although some of them have had to be taken off the program as their dementia has progressed.

The multidisciplinary focus of Planetree is at the crux of creating a nutritional and nurturing long-term care environment. Long-term care must rely heavily upon pharmacists, therapists, and nutritionists who understand the Planetree philosophies. The pharmacist can educate the health team as to which drugs have anorexigenic properties and can suggest possible alternatives. The nutritionist can help the physician eliminate unnecessary dietary restrictions. Therapists can assist in creating an environment conducive to proper nutrition. Time and patience are the necessary ingredients for feeding demented patients who eat slowly and must be reminded to chew and swallow the food.

Choice and involvement are two key components of Planetree. Residents must be allowed to choose the food they eat. Many nursing homes allow the resident councils to choose the menus. Ethnic food choices are an important consideration as well. Delano Regional Medical Center allows residents or their families to call the dietary department with special requests. The staff of the dietary department knows the residents well enough to call them by name and they personally check to see if the food served was eaten by the resident. Notes are kept to ensure that the resident gets the kind of food he or she will eat.

Dennis Sullivan (2000) suggests that "grazing" is an antidote to rigid meal policies and undernutrition in nursing homes. He states, "With advancing age, and especially with cognitive deficits, many older individuals no longer want to adhere to a strict schedule of three meals a day. So if the setting requires that they eat at three specific times or not at all, patients will frequently choose the latter option. This difficulty can be combated by having small quantities of food available at all times for patients to consume as they desire. Allowing patients to 'graze' in this fashion enables them to eat whenever they are hungry and helps ensure that they will receive the proper nutrients."

Blending the nutritional and nurturing aspects of food is an important part of the long-term care environment. Dietitians monitor the resident's nutritional status while the resident's family is encouraged to bring in special foods that the resident enjoys and meets his dietary needs. At Delano Regional Medical Center, the Planetree Café is open twenty-four hours a day for patients and families to cook, or to just sit and chat together. The activities department uses the kitchen in the café for cooking classes and for aroma therapy. The goal is not just to ensure adequate nutrition of the body; it is also to ensure adequate nutrition of the spirit.

Summary

Long-term care should be a comfortable and seamless continuation of a lifetime. Control, choice, a feeling of usefulness, sexuality, happiness, and sadness all have their place. Age or infirmity should not be a signal that what makes us whole as human beings will diminish in any perceptible way. The long-term care environment must be seen as supporting our humanness—and our humaneness.

References

Baro, F., and Dom, R. "Ten Kerselaere: A Contemporary Approach to Geriatric Care in Belgium." [http://www.homemods.org/library/life-span/contemporary.html]. N.d.

Consumer Law Center. "Aging and Health: Long-Term Care: Rights of Nursing Home Residents." [http://wkbn.findlaw.com/health/ltcare/le25_6rights.html]. N.d.

Clarfield, M. "Your Older Patients Also Need Respect." *Nursing Home Medicine: Annals of Long-Term Care Online*, 1998, 6(5). [http://www.mmhc.com/nhm/articles/NHM9805/Commentary.html].

"Elderly Patient Repeatedly Injured in Nursing Home 'Accidents': Negligence, Coincidence or Abuse?" *Brickey v. Concerned Care of Midwest Inc.* 988 S.W. 2d. 592 MO, 1999. [http://www.nursefriendly.com/nursing/clinical.cases/062799.htm].

Fitten, L. J., Morley, J. E., and Gross, P. I. "Depression." *Journal of the American Geriatric Society.* 1989, 37, 459–472.

Fowler, L. K. "Guilt and Making Decisions: Role of Adult Children in Assisting Parents." Ohio State University Fact Sheet. [http://ohioline.osu.edu/flm99/fs05.html]. 1999.

Friends and Relatives of Institutionalized Aged. [http://www.fria.org/html/fria2_guilt.html]. 1998–1999.

Kahn R. "Weight Loss and Depression in a Community Nursing Home." *Journal of the American Geriatric Society*, 1995, *43*, 83.

Kamel, H., Karcic, E., Karcic, A., and Barghouthi, H. "Nutritional Status of Hospitalized Elderly: Differences Between Nursing Home Patients and Community-Dwelling Patients." *Nursing Home Medicine: Annals of Long-Term Care Online*, 2000, 8(3), 33–38.

Langer, E. *Mindfulness*. Cambridge, Mass.: Perseus Publishing, 1989.

Morley, J. E. "Anorexia in Older Persons." *Drugs and Aging*, 1996, 8, 134–152.

"Nursing Home Rehabilitation Stay Proves Terminal: Was Quality of Care Given An Issue?" *Lloyd v. County of Du Page*, 707 N.E. 2d. 1252—IL, 1999. [http://www.lopez1.com/lopez/clinical.cases/071199.htm].

Reiman, S. "The Value of Therapy Dogs in the Long-Term Care Environment." *Nursing Home Medicine: Annals of Long-Term Care Online*, 2000, 8(6). [http://www.mmhc.com/nhm/articles/NHM0006/reiman.html].

Roche, J. "A Personal Look at Long-Term Care: Maintaining a Spiritual Climate." *Nursing Home Medicine: Annals of Long-Term Care Online*, 1997, 5(12). [http://www.mmhc.com/nhm/v5n12.shtml].

Sullivan, D. "Undernutrition in Older Adults." *Nursing Home Medicine: Annals of Long-Term Care Online*, 2000, 8(5).

Takahashi, P. "The Physician's Response to Institutional Mistreatment." *Nursing Home Medicine: Annals of Long-Term Care Online*, 1998, 6(8).

Thomas, B. "Eden Alternative." [http://www.edenalt.com]. 2002.

15

Holistic Hospitals

Planetree on the Spiritual Frontier

Leland Kaiser

Two caterpillars sat on top of a fence post enjoying the beautiful day when a butterfly went flying by. One caterpillar turned to the other and said, "Oh, would you look at that now. You'll never get me up in one of those."

Like the caterpillar, those of us in health care today are taking part in a marvelous transformation that is essential to the field. We are in a process of metamorphosis that we do not fully understand. We are changing form. We are changing at the chrysalis level. When a caterpillar is in the chrysalis stage, it dissolves into a mere liquid. This must be anxiety provoking for the caterpillar. All it has at that point is a hope and a promise that, whereas yesterday it had crawled on its belly, one day it will fly. And that is our promise as well. Today we crawl on our bellies, but one day we shall fly. We must learn to trust the process of transformation, no matter how difficult or anxiety-provoking it may seem. Those of us working in health care have an obligation to be of service in this world, to be bringers of light and hope. Our work is spiritual by its nature, as the Planetree model has acknowledged for decades. The "S" word is a word that we can now use in business and in the corporate world, although we are still a little hesitant to use it in the health care

This chapter is taken from Leland Kaiser's keynote address at the 2001 Planetree annual conference.

world. It is amazing to see our colleagues in the world of business who are beginning to realize that spiritual principles and the highest human values are essential to American capitalism. If the world is to be made better, it will be made better by people with the resources to do so. What we need is capitalism with a conscience.

What we need to learn is a spiritual principle that calls for sharing our abundance with others, because sharing our abundance with others creates greater abundance. America and American capitalism have a socially redemptive mission that we have never accepted. Adam Smith, the economist and philosopher, operated within a moral framework that we have never articulated because, in Smith's time, it was assumed. It was assumed that there was an obligation for those who have to share, in order that all may have. This brought meaning and purpose to the work, imbuing it with an essential spiritual dimension.

Spirituality in Health Care

What we need to see now is spirituality enter health care as its most important dimension. In so doing, it is important that we not confuse spirituality with religion. Mitroff and Benton wrote in *A Spiritual Audit of Corporate America* (1999) that in contrast with conventional religion, spirituality is not formal, structured, or organized, and it is nondenominational and embraces everyone. It is universal and timeless. They note that spirituality is the ultimate source and provider of meaning and purpose in our lives. It expresses the awe we feel in the presence of transcendence. Spirituality recognizes the sacredness of everything, including the very ordinary aspects of everyday life. It can give us a deep sense of interconnectedness with one another, something that our nation had been losing prior to the events of September 11, 2001, and something many of our hospitals and health institutions have not had for some time.

Deep within many of our hospitals and health care centers, that sense of connectedness is missing. We cannot fully serve those who come to us vulnerable and in crisis unless we truly connect with them as individual human beings. Connectivity is consciousness. This is a basic spiritual law. One of the reasons why hospitals become Planetree affiliates is to celebrate the conviction, the dedication, and the passion for a care model that fully embraces the spiritual dimension. But another reason is to connect. Planetree represents a brain trust, a group of people with the potential to transform health care in this nation, on this planet. The Planetree philosophy, when extended a few steps further, is absolute transformation. It is more than a better way of treating patients, more than a better patient facility, more than a way of tapping into the creativity and emotional commitment of health caregivers. It is all of those things and more. It is a synergy that basically changes the culture of the institution and its relationship with its community, its patients, and its employees.

One definition of spirituality is coming into right relationship with all that is, establishing a loving, nurturing, caring relationship. We are in relationship with all that is. We live in a universe of relationships. Anything that we can relate to we share consciousness with and also become that. Planetree's early role has been to refocus our attention on the power of relationships, and, in particular, on the mind-body-spirit relationship essential to healing. What has resulted is a philosophical change, a paradigm shift toward holism in health care. It has opened a door that will never be closed.

We have embarked on a voyage of discovery that has no end— a voyage of discovery that will permanently change each of us in the process, along with our patients, families, and communities. Planetree is one spiritual program that has the power to transform everything it touches. It challenges us to create a spiritual atmosphere in a health facility that says very plainly, *Human beings are multidimensional creatures.* We are multidimensional creatures living in a multidimensional universe. We are much more than our bodies. The greatest mistake of Western medicine has been its attempt to define and then treat multidimensional individuals as bodies only. We are not bodies—we *have* bodies. Like an automobile, the body is a vehicle for our emotional, intellectual, and spiritual selves. Once we understand and accept that we are multidimensional beings, it follows that in order to be effective, our health care has to be multidimensional as well. If we only focus on the patient's body, we are missing three quarters of who that person is. That's a serious omission. Planetree takes us into new dimensions of healing, from the old physics to the new. What we are discovering is that as we treat the patient as a multidimensional being, we suddenly have the ability to heal people in ways we have not had before.

Healing Versus Curing

Much of our current health care is about curing, and curing is scientific. Curing is good. But healing is spiritual, and healing is better, because we can heal many people we cannot cure. Curing people is not always doing them a favor. It simply pushes them to be more creative in developing the next disease they need. One of the most discouraging things we have learned from the field of psychology is the phenomenon of the secondary gain of illness—the discovery that many people need their pathology. Take it away and they have to cast around for a new one, creating in themselves a "revolving door patient." If we do not understand the spiritual dimension of the disease, we do not understand the disease. If our interventions are not spiritual, emotional, and mental as well as physical, we have forfeited a great deal of our therapeutic effectiveness. And if the roots of the disease lie at the spiritual, emotional, or mental level, we will never cure or heal the person by using only physical procedures.

We need four diagnoses on every patient who comes into one of our institutions. We need to ask our hospital chaplains to provide spiritual diagnoses for patients, which are incorporated into the medical record. We need to make the chaplains full partners on the health care team, developing spiritual interventions built around their diagnostic acumen. Unfortunately, many hospital chaplains have no idea how to make a spiritual diagnosis. Many chaplains have not been trained to do a full spiritual assessment. Many chaplains have no idea what the meaning of the disease is in the context of the patient's life, how the disease may be a transformational ally, or how the disease may be an inner teacher and mentor. A disease in one year of an individual's life, if properly understood, may bring about more spiritual growth than a lifetime without disease.

Spiritual Anatomy

The challenge for hospitals is to be in the forefront of healing and spiritual diagnosis. We must understand spiritual anatomy in order to fully help patients. The fundamental impulse that drives each individual is called spirit, or *being*. We are here to incarnate possibilities. We are here to provide the vehicles necessary to manifest spirit on this planet. As spirits, we *are*. As souls, we *know*. As minds, we *think*. As emotions, we *feel*. As bodies, we *act*. If these elements are in alignment or balance, we call that *at one-ment*, or atonement, or, in Eastern traditions, *enlightenment*. It simply means that our multidimensionality is integrated. It means that we are *enspirited*, are whole. It means that energy moves freely among our levels of being.

Once we understand the spiritual anatomy of a person, we can begin to identify the misalignments that might occur. Can a person have sickness of the soul? She can. Can a person have a problem with the mind, thought forms that are obsessive, compulsive, limiting? He can. Can a person have an emotional form that causes tremendous turbulence inside herself? Of course. And what is the body? The body is an indicator of the status of these three levels. That is why treating only the body will never be sufficient, why we must be multidimensional in our healing approaches. The reason Planetree is such an important movement is that Planetree recognizes significant forces that have an impact on the patient, such as the physical environment. We are in correspondence with the

environment that surrounds us. The environment shapes us, limits us, and empowers us. Its impact on us depends on how it is
designed. Planetree designs a space around the patient. When we
make the effort to discover what kind of soil a patient needs in order
to sprout, in order to grow, we are actually gardeners of the human
soul. We are trying to create an environment that evokes potential,
creates possibility, and indicates spirit. Healing architecture is a significant part of that.

Healing Architecture

The most basic question we need to pose in caring for others is this:
Is this a loving act? We are here to nurture each other. Planetree
embodies certain spiritual values, such as feelings, family, friendship, community, connectivity, respect, growth, self-empowerment,
and relationship. All health care facilities should be designed
around those and other values like them. Pose the question *Is this a
loving, nurturing environment?* The qualities of the experience we
want to provide to the patient must be inherent in the patient's
environment. If we want to see a self-empowered patient, we must
build self-empowerment possibilities into the patient's environment.
We respond to the opportunities of the environment within and
around ourselves. The reason Planetree is so powerful is because it is
designed to create an atmosphere, an environment, an ambiance
that stimulates, invokes, pulls out, and encourages empowerment.
We are really in a romantic relationship with our environment; it
is a dance, a symbiotic exchange. We can become empowered or
unempowered by our environment.

When a health care giver walks into the room of a patient, that
health care giver creates an emotional tone, a set of expectations
that are experienced by the patient. When a physician walks into
the patient's room, is there a light that goes from the physician's
heart to the patient's heart? When that physician sits down with
the patient and touches the patient, is there a connection? If that

physician is a spiritual person, he or she will activate the magnetic, or energetic, field of every patient he or she interacts with and will connect heart to heart with every patient, passing a living electrical impulse from him- or herself to the patient. This is the healing moment, the moment of expectation, the moment of connectedness. If the patient's heart is open, if the mind is receptive, what happens is, the soul of the patient communicates with the soul of the doctor and tells the doctor precisely what is needed to feel differently. Intuition is simply connectivity.

We have to know not only what to do but also how to listen. Once the caregiver is perceived by the patient as an ally, once the patient's soul can see that caregiver as a friend, then revelations occur and information is transferred that can happen no other way.

Auditing the Healing Environment

It is essential that the software match the hardware in a healing environment. Even after you have designed the physical environment, and hardwired it with the right values, the people working in it must understand their responsibility in order to be effective. One of the spiritual teachings of Planetree is that we are responsible for the energy we emit at all times. Caregivers should never walk into a patient's room unless they are in a calm, loving, and nurturing frame of mind. A negative emotional state is just as likely to contaminate patients as microbes are. Although the physical environment is very important, it is the spiritual presence within the environment that has the greatest impact on healing, and spirituality may be expressed in many ways in health care settings. The following elements should be evaluated in conducting a spiritual audit of a particular environment:

1. Is there a clear spiritual atmosphere? What statements do the buildings themselves make when you first approach the facility? Do you know that you are on holy ground? Is it a sacred place? Is something different happening here? Can you feel

the energy being created by the people working here? Is powerful, healing, joyful, creative, soulful energy circulating?

2. Does the hospital provide spiritual counsel to families, visitors, and staff members? This may be done within a religious frame of reference, but not necessarily. The aim of the hospital should be to accelerate the spiritual evolution of everyone who steps onto the grounds.

3. Is the hospital open to the unexpected, the unusual, the unexplainable—such as the tumor that was lethal that simply disappears with prayer or meditation? We must offer in our facilities master spiritual healers as well as scientific practitioners. We should be able to say to a patient, "We have the best science and we have the highest spirituality that we can offer. And we will approach you on multiple levels in order to optimize your healing process."

I think the board of trustees in every hospital, by policy, should challenge its management staff, its medical staff, and its nursing staff to look globally to identify any technique, any person, and any process that might have significant value to the patient and to that community. Allow no sacred cows, no taboos. What currently limits us in doing this is our prejudice and our bias. We either have Western medical research evidence of treatment effectiveness, or we don't support it. However, we have yet to see a controlled clinical study explain the myriad medical miracles we hear about regularly.

4. Does the hospital provide spiritual interventions? How often do the physicians give a referral to a spiritual practitioner to help the patient alter his or her consciousness? Spirituality should not be an afterthought, and chaplains should not be seen as auxiliary. They currently are not part of the dominant model of medicine. The challenge is to reach out and create the model developing new spiritual interventions to assist our patients. It has become very clear that prayer can change

patient care outcomes, and healing can occur at a distance. Are we using these modalities to improve the patient experience?

5. Are we creating new mental models, or are we limiting ourselves? All limitations are self-imposed. There are no limitations in the universe.

   A very old story tells of a disciple out for his early morning walk, and as he rounded a bend in the path, he saw his teacher standing in the middle of a river, waist deep. The disciple called out, "Master, what are you doing?" His teacher replied, "I'm looking for something," and the disciple said, "What are you looking for?" "I am looking for water and I can't seem to find it anywhere." At that moment the disciple achieved enlightenment.

   The message is this: If you don't recognize water, you can stand waist deep in a river and die of thirst. Everything we need is already here, but we can't benefit from it if we can't yet see it. Our challenge is to create new mental models for patient care that go beyond what we now define as adequate patient care. We will need to draw outside the lines. We will need to be open-minded but not empty-headed, and we must be willing to look and learn. The people who can help us do this are out there. We have never provided an institutional environment that permits them to think outside the box. So, again, we are limited not by the universe but by our mental model of the universe.

6. How do we use space to alter thinking and behavior? How did the mound builders build the mounds to create the frequencies they created to alter consciousness? What did the cathedral builders know that we have forgotten? What is the power of sacred geometry to resonate with the human soul and activate it? Architecture has three dimensions: the first is functional, the second is aesthetic, and the third is consciousness altering. The great pyramids were designed to be all three. Stonehenge was designed to be all three. Hospitals can be designed to be all three.

7. Are we providing innovative deathing options? There are two great portals in life. One is birth and the other is death. Spirituality is markedly absent at both. As long as we think of birth and death as primarily medical events, we will continue to miss perhaps the most significant opportunities to support the spiritual needs of human beings. Providing deathing services in particular is one of the most humane, compassionate, and loving things we can ever do. No one should ever die alone or in fear. What we do when we help a person die well is to help him or her reconstruct his or her life. Help that person look for things that may need closure before he or she passes on. The goal is to leave with no baggage. Fear can be alleviated by sharing what the process may be like in reassuring terms. Death can be a joyous event. Unfortunately, it is generally just the opposite for patients who die in a hospital. Hospitals are often horrible places to die, where the person is seen as a medical failure and so is not allowed to pass on peacefully.

8. Are courses in spirituality offered for every employee? If we want to have a spiritual hospital, we must provide training in spirituality open to people of all beliefs. We can't create a spiritual environment unless we have a common language, and we won't have a common language unless we have a shared mental model. What if we had spiritual detectors right above the door of the hospital, similar to security at the airport? If your consciousness is not at a high enough level to be helpful to patients and fellow employees, you cannot come through the door. If you phone in to work and say, "I'm vomiting all over the place, I have the flu, and I feel terrible," we'll say, "Stay home; don't come in and expose us." But if you call in and say, "I have a deep and dark depression guaranteed to drag down everybody I come into contact with," we'll say, "You come right on in! We'll never be able to detect you; most of the employees also feel that way." There is something very alarming about this approach.

9. How pervasive are the healing arts and music? Can patients select the music they would like to listen to during surgical procedures? Music appeals to the soul, and we should maximize its healing powers. Healing gardens, meditation paths, and sacred areas in the building should be special places in health care environments.

10. Are complementary and alternative modalities integrated with allopathic medicine? We cannot provide appropriate patient care unless we provide whole person care. There is a need for understanding homeopathic medicine, naturopathy, massage, acupuncture, and many other modalities. We should provide integrative medicine, whether to complement a traditional treatment approach or to replace it. This should depend on the condition.

There is a very simple question to ask to evaluate whether you're offering an appropriate range of therapies. Does every patient who comes into your facility feel better when he or she leaves? When patients come for cancer treatment, do they get a massage, do they sit in the healing garden, do they drink in the music, do they say, "Getting my cancer treatment is a life-transforming experience that elevates my soul"? If that isn't the case, then make the necessary changes. Life is too short, particularly for many cancer patients, to spend time in a treatment environment that isn't truly healing.

In a hospital environment, care can be experiential, interactive, and amusing. Medicine can be art, a scientific form of theater. Its business is providing fundamental soul change through amusement, fun, laughter, and joy. Patch Adams has much to teach us about medical theater: the sense that healing ought to be outrageous and that it ought to be fun. Too many hospitals are bereft of joy by presence or by name. And yet joy and passion create a stir in the universe, a vortex, a disturbance, a time-space displacement that causes forces to move toward the source. The skill is to get out of the way and let them converge. We are magnetic creatures, and we create an actual magnetic storm in a higher dimension. Buddha said that desire *moves*. Joy and passion move. They pull support and resources to them. The creation of an organization with a joyful, passionate culture will cause people to move toward it. Everything we need is already here. We are standing waist deep in it. But like the disciple in the story, at times, we don't recognize it and we need directions.

The business of Planetree is potentiation—creating an environment matched to the person and providing a set of opportunities geared to that person. Many older adults in our communities are woefully underused resources. Hospitals should create *potentiation centers*, where we meet with retirees and say, "You know, you are seventy years old and you've got to face up to the question, what do you want to be when you grow up? You've got thirty more years, use them well." The ultimate strategy for the containment of chronic disease in an aging population is to ensure that every older person is on the path of personal metamorphosis, that their lives make sense, and that they are still unfolding and learning.

In summary, what we need to do is invent the future we want to occupy. We have the potential to take charge of our own evolution. This could not have happened a hundred years ago, or fifty years ago, or even ten years ago. The time is right now. We need to challenge our imagination and our creativity and our beliefs. We need to envision the best of all worlds for our patients, their families, and our employees. If we had all the resources in the world and everyone's permission, what would our institutions look like? Never wait until the time is right; that time never comes. Never wait for the foundation grant or the waiver, and stop excusing nonperformance. There are no excuses. We must do what we can. Get it started. Plant the seed. The rest follows.

Reference

Mitroff, I., and Benton, E. *A Spiritual Audit of Corporate America: A Hard Look at Spirituality, Religion, and Values in the Workplace*. San Francisco: Jossey-Bass, 1999.

16

Transformation and the Future of Health Care

Randall Carter, Susan B. Frampton, Laura Gilpin, Patrick A. Charmel

Like waves upon a beach, trends in every industry emerge continuously, break with some force upon those concerned, alter the landscape of how we operate, and then recede as the next trend appears. Health care has been hit with some tremendous tidal waves over the past several decades, including the deployment of increasingly complex and powerful medical technologies, unanticipated epidemiologic challenges, the growth of managed care and malpractice awards, the rise of health care consumerism, and workforce shortages. Despite these often tumultuous forces, it is absolutely essential that we stay connected to the deeper meaning of what we do. We *care* for people. We don't assemble automobiles, sell insurance, or design clothing, all of which are worthwhile jobs. Caring for people when they are at their most vulnerable is not just a job, it is a mission and a calling. By the very nature of our work, we enter into a personal relationship with our patients and their loved ones, whether we serve their meals, clean their hospital rooms, start their IV lines, or suture their wounds.

Health care is currently in a crisis of meaning. We have lost our focus, distracted by the powerful waves of change that have rendered the work that we do increasingly challenging. We have turned medicine into rocket science, and we have allowed ourselves to be swept up completely by the allure of technology at the expense of simple human dignity. We are turning caring nurses into commodities, encouraging them to jump from one job to another in search of the biggest hiring bonus. Hospital CEOs are decried by their employees as "bean counters," whose priorities have shifted from patients to bottom lines. Patients continue to complain, as they have for the past several decades, of being patronized, being treated like numbers, and being kept in the dark.

Patient-centered care is one approach to bringing health care back to its roots and thus back into balance. It is an approach that has proven successful for the hospitals committed to it. It has the potential to transform an organization's culture when practiced in a consistent and comprehensive manner. It is not, however, a quick fix or a destination an organization arrives at. It is a journey of continually recommitting ourselves to looking at our beliefs and behaviors from the patient's perspective. It is a process of role modeling at all levels. The same personalized, demystified, and humane approach we desire our staff to use with patients and families must also be extended to the staff by managers, to managers by administrators, to nurses by physicians, and so on.

Mahatma Ghandi said, "Be the change you wish to see in the world." This message is particularly relevant today. The way to transform the health care system, which is so often described in terms of the ever-increasing percentage of the gross domestic product (GDP) it absorbs, is ultimately through personal transformation. We must change the way we think about our role in our own personal health, as well as in the health care settings in which we work.

This call for personal responsibility and accountability for our behavior was trumpeted years ago with the advent of the prevention and wellness movement. Diet, exercise, and stress management skills were rightfully heralded as the road to personal health. Third-party payers put forward the concept of capitation partially as an approach to changing the incentives in the system away from treatment after the fact, to preservation of health and well-being.

Although the structure didn't work, the concept was a worthwhile departure from a system in which payment and wellness incentives are often mutually exclusive. In the end, capitation may have been on the right track. However, within the health care system, the provider focus still dominates, and as long as this is the case, prevention and wellness will never be fully embraced and supported. The place of most potential therefore doesn't rest within the medical community, the government, or insurance companies. The place to begin is inside ourselves. As individuals, we have the power to align our behaviors with our values. If we truly value health and well-being, we must pursue it as vigorously as any other important goal in life. We see the powerful signs of this personal pursuit in the tremendous growth in the use of the Internet, as well as in the use of complementary and alternative modalities. Largely self-referred and paying out-of-pocket, individuals remain in control of prevention and treatment options in this parallel health care system.

Hospitals and health care organizations have a wonderful opportunity to support and nurture this growing movement toward personal responsibility and accountability in fundamental ways. In addition, we need to take responsibility for transforming our own organizations by role modeling these same behaviors. Many of those avenues have been presented in the pages of this book. By continually examining our policies, procedures, and practices through the eyes of our patients, we will see the challenges and opportunities that exist for the future. As Leland Kaiser noted in Chapter Fifteen, we can create the future we desire. If we are committed to fostering personal responsibility in our patients, their families, and our employees, we must make the necessary effort. Just as individuals have an enormous capacity to create their own health, hospitals and health care organizations have the ability to transform their culture into one that is truly nurturing and empowering.

Open access to information and education, significant involvement of social support networks, and creation of emotionally, spiritually, and physically healing environments will continue to define the promise of patient-centered care. It is a promise whose fulfillment is no less beneficial to the staff than to patients, their families, and our communities.

Future Vision

Let us imagine where true patient-centered care may take us in the future. Take a moment and put yourself in the patient's shoes.

It was the last day of summer when the diagnosis was delivered to the forty-two-year-old father of two. It seemed ironic timing, given that tomorrow would be the first day of fall. The power of the word *cancer* was heard in his ears but seemed to sink quickly to his now tightening stomach. That was what he noticed, what he felt: the panic growing as he thought, *This can't be happening to me*. The physician sensed the impact of his news and began a gentle but thorough discussion of the treatment options available and the possible progression of the patient's cancer. There was that word again, but after the information and discussion with this compassionate physician, the word began to take shape in a new way in his mind—and in that of his wife. Time was clearly not an ally in their decision-making process, so, together, the patient, family, and physician decided that a rigorous regimen of radiation and chemotherapy would provide the best option for a favorable outcome.

The patient reflected on the amazing series of events. This has been and will continue to be a collaboration of sorts. This disease demands alliances and support from so many, as the needs are both urgent and everywhere all at once—mind, body, and spirit. His care and cure options would need to be diverse. This disease would create many challenges as he progressed through treatment.

He would like to have choices for curing and healing not just for himself, as the patient with cancer, but also for those who loved and supported him, his family. They would make their stand together, putting their trust, faith, and his life in this most human of events. His growing list of needs, concerns, and life changes made him dizzy. Where do you go to receive caring for such diverse needs? Is there a place designed with the intention necessary to meet the needs of curing and healing while supporting the spiritual and intellectual needs of patients, families, and those who love and support them?

Organizations that practice patient-centered care are the guides to many of the answers to these questions. And as providence would provide for this patient, a cancer center that embraces patient-centered philosophies is available in his region. The center offers the best of technology as well as opportunities for choices and support that come from traditional healing practices. This facility, built with the full intention to meet the needs of patients, families, and caregivers, offers a diversity of tools and access points for caring. It provides to health care the most recent guidepost of what the future of the patient and his family experiences could be.

The patient's first visit to the center is an experience of intense anxiety and fear. In preparation, he has read the literature provided in advance by his physician, has consulted the resource library, and has conducted his own Internet research. But the first step this morning is to leave his familiar home, get into his car, and begin the journey toward the unknown details of his treatments, which assails his confidence. He continues with support and a gentle touch from his son as he leaves for school. "I'll be thinking of you, Dad. We love you and we'll get through this. Our family is strong together."

Upon arrival at the cancer facility, he and his wife are struck by the welcome they receive from the staff and volunteers and by the warmth of the environment. Something is different here. A feeling of calmness and purposeful nurturing and support is present. "This is a beginning" says the nurse coordinator, and the words seem to echo in his ears. They have just met but the impact is immediate. She has a ready smile and a depth of belief and caring that makes a difference simply through her presence.

"At the center," she continues, "you will have a number of choices available to meet your needs for mind, body, and spirit." She begins a walking tour of the campus, pausing to introduce each feature and the team members and their respective roles in creating this healing environment. "We have a number of quiet meditative spaces and gardens for your use," she says, as they near something unexpected—a labyrinth located conveniently in front of the center. "It's a wonderful place for our patients and their support network to gather together their spiritual resources prior to and after treatment here at the center, and it's open and available twenty-four hours a day."

The tour continues as they reenter the building, walking past a cascading water feature that calms and connects to this region's geography, bringing the familiarity of home into this place of healing. "What is the 'center for mindfulness'?" the patient's wife asks as she looks at the muted entry sign. "That's our next stop," the nurse explains. "This center, with its spa and meditation garden, is designed to nurture the body, mind, and spirit and is for use by both patients and their families. In addition to sauna and Jacuzzi areas, this part of the facility provides treatment space for acupuncture and massage practitioners and is available for patients as they move through the treatment process." The tour moves through a private corridor to the technical side of the care provided. The nurse explains that the highest-quality technological treatment is provided here, with an equal focus on the high-touch aspects of caring. The rooms are well appointed and homelike to the degree possible in this environment. Things are well kept and clean, and for the most part, the anxiety is lowered by a focus on interior details instead of on the technology. Great attention has been paid to design places so as to temporarily store equipment out of sight of the patient, but the equipment is in ready proximity for the caregivers and technicians. As they leave this technical area, they are struck by the calm and confident spirit of this center and its difference—a pleasant and important surprise.

As the facility tour ends, they return to the center's patient and family library, and the nurse answers questions about the upcoming treatment process and provides additional resources from the library's collection. The patient and his wife try to gather in every detail and are concerned that they may have forgotten to ask important questions. They ask, "Is there anything else we should know?" There is a smile now with the warmth of a trusted guide. It arrives on the nurse's face as she says, "Yes, we have a number of support activities available for you and your family. They are offered to you as choices to augment and enhance your treatment experience. We have traditional support groups that gather during the month as well as programs on journaling, *prayer ties* from the Lakota tradition, drumming circles, yoga, and tai chi." As she reaches for each of their hands, she says, "Our goal is simply to provide you with what

312 PUTTING PATIENTS FIRST

you need as you go through this journey, whether that
need is for your mind, your body, or your spirit. We are
your partners in this process. We will be here." With
that, she points to the patient lobby area, indicating a
man and his wife who are receiving shoulder and neck
massages from the facility's therapist, and she says, "Be
sure you have a massage. When you come in for treatment, it really makes a difference." The patient and his
wife rise and thank their new friend and express their
gratitude for her time and introduction to the facility
and, most important, to the caring nurses, physicians,
and staff members who make this experience possible.
They turn toward the door to leave. As they walk past
the large window looking out onto the restful waterfall,
they notice for the first time a carving on the surface of
the stone closest to the window. "That's a water guardian,"
a voice from behind them says. They turn to see a smiling volunteer moving toward them, and as he introduces
himself, he continues: "There are eleven of those petroglyphs on the falls. They are sacred to the Native Americans of this area. They believe that these images have
the power to protect and heal those in their presence.
Found along the rivers of this region, they were created
thousands of years ago. It just seems important for them
to be here to continue their vigil for those who journey
to this place of healing."

The patient helps his wife into the car and then
moves slowly to his door and pauses, looking at the
changing leaves of the sycamores that welcomed him to
the center. He reflects on his journey these past few days
and it is autumn, and with it comes not only the falling
of the leaves but also the promise of renewal. The car
door shuts.

Summary

The scenario above is not a fantasy. It is a reality in one small Planetree hospital, and if it can happen in one hospital, it can happen anywhere. We cannot wait for insurance companies, the government, or other outside agencies to create this reality, anymore than patients can expect quick fixes for conditions better treated with personal lifestyle changes. The answers need to come from within. We *are* health care, and so we cannot expect someone else to transform the system for us. Every individual in health care can participate in providing the very best experience for patients, thus taking responsibility for being a part of the transformation. This has been Planetree's essential mission: to bring this vision into reality by empowering and engaging every patient, family member, volunteer, and employee in the endeavor.

Planetree Alliance Member List

The Planetree Alliance is a growing network of hospitals and health care organizations using the Planetree patient-centered model of care. Examples of innovative practices, approaches, and programs included throughout this book were drawn from many of the organizations listed here.

ALBERT EINSTEIN MEDICAL CENTER
5501 Old York Road
Philadelphia, PA 19141

ALEGENT HEALTH
Bergan Mercy Medical Center
Mercy Hospital
Immanuel Medical Center
Midlands Community Hospital
1010 North 96th Street, Suite 200
Omaha, NE 68114

ALLIANCE COMMUNITY HOSPITAL
264 East Rice Street
Alliance, OH 44601

AURORA BAYCARE MEDICAL CENTER
P.O. Box 8900
Green Bay, WI 54308–8900
2845 Greenbrier Road
Green Bay, WI 54311

AURORA MEDICAL CENTER–MARITOWOC
5000 Memorial Drive
Two Rivers, WI 54241

AVERY HEALTH CARE SYSTEM
Charles A. Cannon Jr. Memorial Hospital
434 Hospital Drive
P.O. Box 787
Linville, NC 28646

BANNER HEALTH SYSTEM
Desert Samaritan Medical Center
Good Samaritan Regional Medical Center
Page Hospital
Valley Lutheran Hospital
1441 North 12th Street
Phoenix, AZ 85006

BERKSHIRE MEDICAL CENTER
725 North Street
Pittsfield, MA 01201

BETH ISRAEL MEDICAL CENTER
First Avenue at 16th Street
3 Dazian Pavilion
New York, NY 10003

CATSKILL REGIONAL MEDICAL CENTER
P.O. Box 800
68 Harris-Bushville Road
Harris, NY 12742-0800

COLUMBIA MEMORIAL HOSPITAL
2111 Exchange Street
Astoria, OR 97103

DELANO REGIONAL MEDICAL CENTER
1401 Garces Highway
P.O. Box 460
Delano, CA 93215

FAUQUIER HOSPITAL
500 Hospital Drive
Warrenton, VA 20186

FORUM HEALTH
Trumbull Memorial Hospital
Northside Medical Center
3530 Bellmont Avenue, #7
Youngstown, OH 44504

GOOD SAMARITAN HEALTH SYSTEM
10 East 31st Street
Kearney, NE 68847

GREENVILLE HOSPITAL SYSTEM
Allen Bennett Hospital
Greenville Memorial Hospital
Hillcrest Hospital
701 Grove Road
Greenville, SC 29605

GRIFFIN HOSPITAL
130 Division Street
Derby, CT 06418

HACKENSACK UNIVERSITY MEDICAL CENTER
30 Prospect Avenue
Hackensack, NJ 07601

HIGHLINE COMMUNITY
HOSPITAL SYSTEM
Highline Community Hospital
Highline Specialty Center
16251 Sylvester Road, SW
Burien, WA 98166

HUDSON RIVER HEALTHCARE, INC.
1037 Main Street
Peekskill, NY 10566

KANE COMMUNITY HOSPITAL
North Fraley Street
P.O. Box 778
Kane, PA 16735

LAKELAND HOSPITAL NILES
31 North St. Joseph Avenue
Niles, MI 49120

LITTLETON ADVENTIST HOSPITAL
7700 South Broadway
Littleton, CO 80122

LONGMONT UNITED HOSPITAL
1950 Mountain View Avenue
Longmont, CO 80501

LOUISE OBICI MEMORIAL HOSPITAL
2800 Godwin Boulevard
Suffolk, VA 23434-8038

MID-COLUMBIA MEDICAL CENTER
1700 East 19th Street
The Dalles, OR 97058

NORTH VALLEY HOSPITAL
6575 Highway 93 South
Whitefish, MT 59937

NORTHERN WESTCHESTER HOSPITAL CENTER
400 East Main Street
Mount Kisco, NY 10549

NORTHSIDE HOSPITAL
1000 Johnson Ferry Road, NE
Atlanta, GA 30342-1611

PORTER ADVENTIST HOSPITAL
2525 South Downing Street
Denver, CO 80210-5876

SAINT JOHN'S REGIONAL MEDICAL CENTER
2727 McClelland Avenue
Joplin, MO 64804-1694

SAINT JOSEPH HOSPITAL AND HEALTH CENTER
1907 West Sycamore Street
P.O. Box 9010
Kokomo, IN 46904

SAINT JOSEPH REGIONAL MEDICAL
CENTER–MISHAWAKA
215 West Fourth Street
Mishawaka, IN 46544

SHANDS AT AGH
801 Southwest 2nd Avenue
Gainesville, FL 32601

SHARP CORONADO HOSPITAL
AND HEALTHCARE CENTER
250 Prospect Place
Coronado, CA 92133

SHAWANO MEDICAL CENTER
309 North Bartlette Street
Shawano, WI 54166

UNIVERSITY OF NORTH CAROLINA
HEALTH CARE SYSTEM
101 Manning Street
Chapel Hill, NC 27514

UPPER CHESAPEAKE HEALTH
Fallston General Hospital
Harford Memorial Hospital
500 Upper Chesapeake Drive
Bel Air, MD 21014

VA HEALTHCARE NETWORK 2
UPSTATE NEW YORK
VA Medical Center–Bath
VA Medical Center–Canandaigua

VA *Medical Center–Syracuse*
VA *Medical Center–Batavia*
VA *Medical Center–Albany*
113 Holland Avenue
G.E.B.H.
Albany, NY 12208

VALLEY VIEW HOSPITAL
1906 Blake Avenue
Glenwood Springs, CO 81601

WARREN MEMORIAL HOSPITAL
1000 North Shenandoah Avenue
Front Royal, VA 22630

WELLMONT HEALTH SYSTEM
Wellmont Bristol Regional Medical Center
1 Medical Park Boulevard
Bristol, TN 37620
Wellmont Holston Valley Medical Center
130 West Ravine Road
Kingsport, TN 37660
Wellmont Lonesome Pine Hospital
1990 Holton Avenue East
Big Stone Gap, VA 24219
Wellmont Hawkins County Memorial Hospital
851 Locust Street
Rogersville, TN 37857

WESLEY VILLAGE
580 Long Hill Avenue
Shelton, CT 06484

WILLIAMSBURG COMMUNITY HOSPITAL
301 Monticello Avenue
Box 8700
Williamsburg, VA 23185-2833

WINDBER MEDICAL CENTER
600 Somerset Avenue
Windber, PA 15963

Name Index

Subject Index

nutrition programs for, 85–86; and
self-management programs, 65;
and social connectedness, 6
Helplessness, 276, 281
Highline Community Hospital, 34,
41, 43, 59
Hippocratic oath, 119, 236
Hogan, ceremonial, 102
Holism, xxxii, 90, 91, 101, 153, 165.
See also Spiritual entries
Holistic hospitals, awareness in, and
approaches of, 293–304
Home-based working options, 225, 232
Homeopathic medicine, 148
Hopelessness, 64
Hospice, 102
Hospital Food, 72, 87
Hospital for Sick Children, 251
Hospital incentives, 267, 306–307
Hospital smell, 83
Hospitality model, 76, 80
Hospital-like environment, 117
Hospitals for a Healthy Environment
(H2E), 259–260
Housekeepers, 7, 11, 217, 275
Hudson River Healthcare, 59
Human interaction: design support-
ing, 171–172; in food service, 82;
importance of, overview of, 3–5;
in long-term care, 265, 273–274;
needed types of, 10–13, 17–23;
roles of, 5–9, 15–17; supporting,
organizational transformation for,
23–25. *See also specific interactions*
Human Resources (HR) department,
221, 223
Human touch, importance of, 105.
See also Massage therapy
Humor, xxxii, 139, 140, 142, 155
Humor carts, 139
Hype and popularity, 28

I

Illness: educational opportunity in,
41; secondary gain of, phenomenon
of, 296

Imams, 99
Immigrant populations, serving, 32, 37
Incentives, hospital, 267, 306–307
Incineration, 236–237, 242, 244–245,
246, 248
Indoor air pollution, 249; avoiding,
252, 253–258, 262
Industrialized society, environmental
impact of, 235–236
Industry evolution, concept relevant
to, 206
Industry shifts, 195–197, 206
Industry size, 213, 236
Industry status quo, commitment to,
203
Industry trends, xxxiv, 153, 159, 305
Infant massage, 113
Infectious disease and global warming,
240
Infectious waste, 246
Information access: to CAM, xxxi,
46, 208; and consumerism, 197;
need for, xxvii, 27–29; summary on,
48; ways of providing, 30–47. *See
also* Consumer health libraries and
resource centers; Open-chart poli-
cies; Patient and family education
Information explosion, xxxiv, 28, 31
Information withholding: from
patients, 27–28; from staff, 19–20
Inpatient settings and CAM integra-
tion, 153, 157, 158–159
Insomnia, 157
Institute for Family-Centered Care,
65, 67
Institute of Medicine, 40, 48, 51, 68,
199
Institutional look of meals, transforming, 76–77
Institutional review boards, 100
Insurance coverage, lack of, 114, 149,
152, 158
Insurance, malpractice, 200
Insurance plans, long-term care, 267
Integrated devices and documenta-
tion systems, benefits of, 232

Sincerity of management, 16
Skilled nursing facilities, 266, 267
Social connectedness, definition of, 6
Social isolation, 5, 6, 279
Social issues, recognizing, 91–92
Social support, effects of, 5–6, 7. See
    also Family and friend involvement;
    Support groups
Socialization, encouraging, in long-
    term care, 265, 278, 279, 280, 281
Software, patient assessment, 110
Soil pollution, 235
Solar energy, 261
Solariums, 284
Solid waste production and disposal,
    240, 245–246, 248, 251, 261–262
Sound factors in facility design,
    182–183
Southern Illinois Healthcare News,
    250, 264
Spas/Jacuzzis, 174, 178, 283
Special diets, 77–78, 290
Special needs, sensitivity to, 82, 274.
    See also Cultural sensitivity
Special procedures, music during,
    141
Spirit-body-mind relationship, atten-
    tion to. See Holism
Spirits, understanding, 297
Spiritual anatomy, 297–298
Spiritual assessment, 94–95, 97
Spiritual atmosphere, evaluating,
    299–300
Spiritual Audit of Corporate America, A
    (Mitroff and Benton), 294
Spiritual audits, 299–303
Spiritual care: case study of, 100–101;
    design supporting, 188; in long-
    term care, 275–276; model pro-
    grams of, 101–103; overview of,
    89–90; practices in, 94–103; train-
    ing in, 91, 101, 302
Spiritual caregivers, faith-based. See
    Pastoral caregivers
Spiritual counseling, 96–97, 300
Spiritual diagnoses, 296–297

Spiritual interventions, 96–99,
    300–301
Spiritual operating principles,
    293–294
Spiritual presence, auditing environ-
    ment for, 299–303
Spiritual screening, 94–95
Spiritual values, 298–299
Spirituality: in health care operations,
    294–296; as an inner resource,
    exploring workings of, 93–94;
    overview of, 89–90; training on, 89,
    302; working definitions of, 92–93
Spirituality and Health, 89
Staff camaraderie, 16
Staff communication: and participa-
    tion, 19–22, 24; in recruitment and
    retention, 202, 215, 216, 218–219,
    221, 225
Staff decision making, 24, 218,
    222–223, 275
Staff disenchantment, xxvi–xxvii
Staff empowerment, 24
Staff gender, 222
Staff interaction, encouraging, xxx,
    46, 82, 171–172, 177, 283
Staff majority, 13
Staff massage, 19, 108, 112–113,
    113–114
Staff, medical. See Physician entries
Staff mind-set, 53, 54
Staff orientation, 225–229
Staff participation, 19–22, 24
Staff recruitment. See Recruitment
    and retention
Staff reductions, 196
Staff retention. See Recruitment and
    retention
Staff retreats, 24, 53, 101, 206, 207,
    229, 275–276
Staff role playing, 67
Staff salaries and wages. See Compen-
    sation
Staff satisfaction: and hospital cafe-
    terias, 80; interactions contribut-
    ing to, 17–23; key employment